Foreword to the second edition by the Minister for Health and Social Services

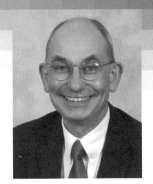

I am delighted to present this second and revised edition of the Good Practice Guide originally produced by the former Innovations in Care. Published halfway through the Assembly sponsored programme to implement the Guide in all Trusts in Wales, this new edition has more practical examples of good practice, an excellent chapter on the role of patients within this work and more guidance on the people aspects of change.

During the last year, we have seen welcome improvements in waiting times across Wales and we have seen evidence of systems changing so that improvements can be sustained. The task is now to ensure that these improvements become integral parts of service delivery. Patients of NHS Wales have the right to expect patient focused, responsive services.
We know that this can be actioned through better use of staff and resources as advocated by this guide.

In 'Designed for Life' I have set out a vision for NHS Wales and its development over the next 10 years. I expect to see the NHS become the jewel in the crown of public services in Wales. The National Leadership and Innovation Agency for Healthcare will provide vital support for the NHS in achieving these goals. This guide, which is already being adapted for use in other home countries, is an excellent example of that support in action.
I commend the Guide to the NHS in Wales, to its staff and patients.

Dr Brian Gibbons AM
Minister for Health and Social Care

Foreword to the first edition by former Minister for Health and Social Services, Jane Hutt AM

I am pleased that Innovations in Care has been able to produce this guide and make it available to all organisations within NHS Wales. It sets out a vision for sustainable good practice within NHS Wales. Its ultimate aim is to create a single integrated approach to all contacts between a patient and a trust. It addresses the interests both of healthcare professionals and patients.

"The importance of patients' voices is recognised as being centrally important in the drive for service improvement...

"Attention will be paid to involving patients more in decisions about their care and in providing adequate evidence to help patients make informed decisions"

(Improving the Health in Wales, 2001)

It is hoped that this document will act as a catalyst for making this happen. It is aimed at all staff who are in a position to be pro-active in introducing improvements and change within their organisation.

The Review of Health and Social Care, advised by Derek Wanless made clear that the current position in NHS Wales is not sustainable, that hospital waiting lists are unacceptably long, that there needs to be integrated thinking across health and social care boundaries, and that best practice should be constantly encouraged.

This document helps respond to those challenges. It has a clear aim to improve the experience of patients and use resources better. It is innovative, offering a fundamental rethinking of the way in which we provide inpatient and outpatient services. This offers an improved service everywhere as an alternative to simply making patients travel to get a better service. Better communication with patients is at the heart of this approach.

As the Wanless report says, demand will always outstrip supply; increasing the capacity of the acute sector will not on its own solve the problem of demand; alternatives are needed. This document gives alternatives; for example looking at how waiting lists are prioritised and questioning whether some referrals and appointments are actually necessary, using better patient communication as the catalyst.

The need to ensure that high quality, accurate and complete information is being shared between a patient and NHS organisations has become more apparent following the highly publicised Climbié, Bristol Royal Infirmary, and Alder Hey scandals.

Patient involvement is vital as patients know best what they want from their service.

The Key Points

1. Overall aim is to ensure patient appointments reflect clinical priority. Patients will be seen in chronological order and given an opportunity to choose a convenient date. This will minimise non-attendances and cancellations.

2. Patient access to hospital services will match standards and expectations, improving patient satisfaction.

3. Communication between hospital, patients and GPs will be better.

4. Patient cancellations and non-attendance rates will be reduced by promoting shared agreements between patients and the trust and applying new ways of communicating with patients.

5. Hospital cancellations will be reduced by applying better management practices and working with staff and patients.

6. Waiting times, and the number of patients waiting, will be reduced by implementing long term capacity planning methods

This document reaffirms the importance that the Welsh Assembly Government and the Innovations in Care team attach to finding innovative ways to eliminate the suffering and uncertainty that accompanies long waits for treatment.

Significant changes are occurring across the NHS within the United Kingdom, and it is hoped that this document will promote the same success as similar programmes implemented by our colleagues in England, Scotland and Northern Ireland.

The Wanless report has highlighted the need for urgent reform and the need to modernise. Innovations in Care must continue to find innovative ways of dealing with the problem.

NHS organisations should adopt the practices described in this report.

Jane Hutt
Minister for Health and Social Services
July 1999 - January 2005

This document was written and edited by members of the National Leadership and Innovation Agency for Healthcare, Elective Services Team (Asiantaeth Genedlaethol Arweiniad ac Arloesoldeb dros Ofal Iechyd, Gwasanaethau Dewisol).

Allan Cumming   Dominique Morton   Claire Lloyd

Mike Fealey   Nia Richards   Alan Willson

Chapter 4 was written by members of the patient partnership group for the Guide to Good Practice Programme. (See page 88).

Acknowledgements
This guide represents tools and techniques developed in Wales, England, the United States and New Zealand. It draws on the work of many people in many organisations.

We would like to particularly acknowledge the work being done by the Modernisation Agency in England, The Centre for Change and Innovation in Scotland and the Institute of Healthcare Improvement in the United States.

Particular thanks go to the Modernisation Agency Capacity and Demand group and the work of Dr Kate Silvester.

Relationships to previous documents
This policy document replaces previous documents issued by Innovations in Care. This includes the following documents:

Expected Standards for Waiting List Management in Wales (November 2000).

Achieving the Expected Standards for Waiting List Management in Wales: Self Assessment Toolkit (December 2000).

Meeting the Expected Standards for Waiting List Management in Wales (October 2001).

A Guide to Good Practice: Outpatients Diagnostics Therapies and Elective Surgery (October 2003, March 2004).

An electronic copy of this guide can be downloaded from: www.nliah.wales.nhs.uk

Contents

Who should use this guide?

This document addresses two unacceptable issues: insufficient recognition of the importance of patient centred care, and a poor use of existing staff and resources. Both could be alleviated within the resources currently available to the NHS in Wales. This guide is based upon evidence of what works — some examples from Wales, some from other countries — and using the guide will result in significant improvement in service delivery. It should be used by all NHS Staff who are involved in the management of patients.

This includes senior Trust management, outpatient managers, theatre managers, and managers of clinical services. It also includes clinicians: medical and nursing staff, professions allied to medicine, and diagnostic staff.

How to use this guide

The document contains examples of good practice, and tools and techniques. Each tool may be used independently, or as a part of an overall service improvement programme.

Some chapters (especially chapters 2 and 3) contain specific guidance for implementing systems recommended by the National Leadership and Innovation Agency for Healthcare and the Welsh Assembly Government. The remainder contains tools that may be useful in a wide range of improvement projects.

Aims and principles

The Welsh Assembly Government is committed to ensuring that people receive speedy treatment in the NHS. Improving Health in Wales states that the aim of the NHS in Wales is to have *'waiting times for elective treatment that are as good as, if not better than, the best in the UK'*[1]. To achieve better waiting times will mean a fundamental rethinking of the way in which inpatient and outpatient services are provided. This document will help NHS staff achieve those goals.

The Guide to Good Practice was first published by the Innovations in Care Team in October 2003. A reprint was published as a workbook for the Implementing the Guide to Good Practice Programme in March 2004. During 2004 and 2005 extra sections were added to the Workbook. This edition of the Guide brings together the original publication, along with the additional sections, as well as a substantial rewriting and expansion of sections related to prioritisation and process mapping.

This edition is published by the National Leadership and Innovation Agency for Healthcare (Asiantaeth Genedlaethol Arweiniad ac Arloesoldeb dros Ofal Iechyd). The Agency was formed by the merger of Innovations in Care and the Centre for Health Leadership Wales in November 2004, and has responsibility for the work formerly done by those two organisations.

The aim of this document is that all contacts between patients and a Trust are managed within a single integrated approach, and it provides tools to achieve that end.

In a patient focused service, there should be a standard way of making appointments. The process for the patient should be the same whether for new or follow-up out-patient appointments, for day treatment, investigations, elective inpatient or day case interventions.

There are six core principles behind this document:

1 Patient choice

The patient should always be offered reasonable choice in their appointment. Choice means that the patient can choose the location, the date and time, and the consultant.

The *reasonable* nature of the choice means that choice may be limited to those locations where clinics and/or theatre sessions are held, dates and times that clinics and lists are scheduled, and consultants or other staff that are qualified to perform the procedure or see the patient.

Reasonable patient choice means that where an option is available, the patient has the right to choose that option.

> **GOOD PRACTICE POINT**
>
> **Standard Integrated Process**
>
> *There should be a standard way of making all appointments within NHS Trusts. The process should cover new and follow-up outpatient appointments, physiotherapy, endoscopy, and radiology. The same principles and processes should also apply for elective inpatient and day case events.*

1 *Improving the Health in Wales: A Guide for the NHS with its partners.* Welsh Assembly Government, 2001

2 An agreed appointment

The patient will have the opportunity to agree the date and time of an appointment with the Trust, either in person or by telephone.

In no case should an appointment time be notified to a patient who has not been involved in the choosing of the date and time.

3 Separate patient choice from Trust performance

There will be times where patient choice conflicts with the Trust's efforts to meet targets or operate efficiently. Patients may choose a date that exceeds Trust waiting time targets.

The key principle in such a case is that patient choice is respected but that Trust performance is not adversely affected.

Where patient choice is the only reason that a target is breached, then that patient should not be included in performance measures.

4 Patients will be treated in turn within agreed clinical priority

Patients are usually assigned a clinical priority when a referral is received or they are placed on a waiting list. Wherever practicable, patients should be seen in priority order.

Within each clinical priority, patients should be seen in the order that they were placed on the list unless the condition or circumstances suggest otherwise, or good management suggests an earlier appointment.

5 An integrated set of policies

Trusts should have an integrated waiting list policy.

The policy should reflect procedures across all working practices in the Trust, and should link into other Trust policies such as patient record policies, admission and discharge policy, staff leave policy, cancelled operations policy and cancer minimum standards policy.

The integrated waiting list policy must include a statement which describes the purpose behind it. Trust clinicians and managers and the Local Health Board (LHB) must all be involved in the development, on-going review, and administration of the policy. The policy must be signed off by the Trust Board Executive accountable for waiting list management, and be formally adopted by the Trust Board.

6 Trusts should be aiming to continually improve services

What is best practice in Wales today will be standard practice tomorrow. Trusts should never see good practice as a final goal.

Trusts must continually improve services, always seeking to make today's best practice normal, and to develop new standards for tomorrow.
'Best Practice' is a commitment to continuous improvement across the organisation.

GOOD PRACTICE POINT

Targets and Goals

Goals set within a service should be aspirational and meaningful to patients. As a long term goal waiting times for outpatients of six days or less, and waits for elective surgery of six weeks or less, should be aimed for.

Targets

This guide will help Trusts achieve the targets set by the Welsh Assembly Government, the NHS Regional Offices, and the SaFF process. These targets will move on from year to year as services improve, and are not included in this document. However, annual SaFF targets should not be seen as the best level of service that the NHS will ever be able to provide.

The National Leadership and Innovation Agency for Healthcare recommends that services set long term goals that relate to what the patient wants. These internal goals may be different to Assembly and SaFF targets. They should be ambitious and guide action for improvement.

Internal targets or goals should be seen as the ultimate point to aim for — the point at which to say 'This is a service that meets all the needs of our patients, and which has achieved waiting times that cannot be improved'.

The NLIAH recommends that services set an internal goal of a six day maximum wait for outpatients, and a six week maximum wait for a procedure. The NHS may not achieve this goal in the short or even the medium term, but until the NHS delivers a service that meets these goals, it should continue striving to improve.

Improvement goals

The NLIAH recommends that improvement efforts focus on six key goals. These are taken from a report on the state of American healthcare[1]. We believe that these six areas of improvement apply equally to the NHS.

Safety

Healthcare is not safe, either in absolute terms or in comparison to other industries or activities. The NHS must continually strive to make healthcare and hospitals safer for patients, and Trusts should work closely with the National Patient Safety Agency to achieve this improvement.

Effectiveness

The NHS must continually work to improve the effectiveness of clinical services:

■ Administrative processes and procedures must ensure that the right patient receives care from the right professional in the right fashion and location.

■ Where there is evidence that a procedure or treatment is effective, that treatment must be offered to those that need it.

■ Where there is no evidence that a procedure or treatment is effective, the procedure or treatment should not be offered.

Patient Centredness

All care should be centred around the patient, with the patient being an active participant in the process. This means that decisions about care should directly involve the patient, that full information is provided at all stages, and that the patient is able to be an equal in all decisions made.

Patient Centredness involves more than the treatment process. Improvement efforts must include patients as active members of the team. Groups that set policy should involve patients. Patient views and concerns should be incorporated into all stages of any redesign of services.

1 *Crossing the Quality Chasm.* Committee on the Quality of Health Care in America, 2001

Timeliness

Care should be provided in a timely fashion. This means that waiting time targets within the Trust should be based on what the patient considers reasonable. This is why the NLIAH recommends six days as the long term goal for outpatient and diagnostic procedures, and six weeks for day case and inpatient procedures.

Timeliness also applies to the administrative process. Standards should be set for time taken to respond to letters, and for process times within the Trust. Administrative procedures should not waste staff time, and workflow through the clinical system should happen as quickly and smoothly as possible.

Efficiency

Money wasted in the health system could have been used to treat patients. Trusts have an obligation to provide patient care in a way that is as efficient as possible, reducing nonproductive practices and waste to a minimum. It is also true that it is hard to build a quality organisation that does not recognise the importance of quality across all aspects of its performance. It is not easy to deliver high quality clinical care in an environment that does not practice quality in administrative practices.

Equity

We should be providing care fairly, ensuring that factors such as social background, race or location do not reduce access to care.

What is the cost of poor quality?

Most of the time, improvement processes in the NHS do not measure efficiency or money saved. It is sometimes assumed that improvement work is about increased quality, and that increased quality means increased cost. This is not the case. In a high proportion of situations quality can be improved by removing wasteful processes, thereby reducing, not increasing, costs.

The NHS must start to measure cost savings as part of the improvement process. It must show that the work of improving patient care is about improved quality by reducing waste, and must start putting figures on the cost of that waste. This will show the real cash value of innovation work, and make it easier to fund future work.

Good practice points

There are a number of points of good practice throughout this guide. They appear in boxes within the text. Here we present the points as a summary of good practice.

Standard Integrated Process
There should be a standard way of making all appointments within NHS Trusts. The process should cover new and follow-up outpatient appointments, physiotherapy, endoscopy, and radiology. The same principles and processes should also apply for elective inpatient and day case events. page 1

Targets and Goals
Goals set within a service should be aspirational and meaningful to patients. As a long term goal waiting times for outpatients to six days or less, and waits for elective surgery of six weeks or less, should be aimed for. page 2

Improvement Goals
NHS Trusts should aim to continually improve services to patients. Improvement should focus on:

- Patient **Safety**;
- Services **centred on patients**;
- **Efficient** provision of services;
- Provision of clinically **effective** services;
- Services provided in a **timely** way;
- **Equity** of access.

page 3

Waiting Lists
A patient should only be placed on a waiting list when all preconditions for treatment have been met. As a test, no patient should be active on a surgical waiting list unless the procedure could be performed tomorrow if the appropriate resources were available. page 19

Validation
On all waiting lists, validation should be undertaken at the point the patient is placed on the list, then at six months, and again at 12 months. In the exceptional circumstance where a patient waits over 12 months, validation should be repeated at 18 months and then at six monthly intervals. page 29

Prioritisation
Clinical prioritisation increases waiting times for lower clinical priority patients. Where clinical prioritisation is necessary, the fewest number of categories should be used. The National Leadership and Innovation Agency for Healthcare recommends using only two categories of prioritisation (Urgent and Routine). Points-based systems, or systems with many degrees of urgency, are not recommended. page 35

> **GOOD PRACTICE EXAMPLE**
> **Examples of Improvement Across Wales**
>
> *Throughout the guide, boxes like this contain examples of improvement initiatives from Welsh Trusts and other parts of the NHS.*
> *These examples are not necessarily 'best' practice, but they are included as examples of Trusts looking at the service they provide to patients and saying 'How can we improve?'*

Primary Targeting Lists

Wherever patients are being selected from a waiting list, the waiting list must be prioritised and sorted. Waiting lists should be sorted first by clinical priority, and then by the date the patient was added to the list. Patients should be removed from the top of the list: longest waiting 'urgent' patients first, shortest waiting 'routine' patients last. page 42

Patient Focused Booking

All appointments where the patient attends the Trust should be booked. The key requirements of patient focused booking are that the patient is directly involved in negotiating the appointment date and time, and that no appointment is made more than six weeks into the future. page 53

Generic Referrals and Pooling

Referrals into Trusts should be pooled within specialities. Referrals to a specific consultant by a GP should only be accepted when there are specific clinical requirements, or stated patient preference. page 55

Preoperative Assessment

Preoperative assessment should be undertaken six weeks prior to surgery, and should be booked using partial booking. Preoperative assessment allows both staff and patient to check suitability for anaesthetic and surgery, agree the booking date for surgery, and organise discharge arrangements. page 82

Building partnerships with patients

Patients should be involved as partners at all levels of the improvement process. Patients should be represented on all project teams, and patient views sought on proposed solutions. It is not possible to build a quality service without an active partnership with patients. page 94

Copying Letters to Patients

All communications between health professionals should be copied to the patient. Patients must be given the right to opt out of receiving letters. Good practice is to write all letters to the patient, and copy the letter to the other health professional. page 105

Managing Capacity and Demand

Staff managing services in Trusts must have a clear understanding of the capacity of their service, the activity levels provided by the service, the demand on the service, and the backlog of work in the system. For non-outpatient work some element of casemix must be incorporated into the measures used. page 109

GOOD PRACTICE POINT

Improving Theatre Utilisation

All Trust should complete the Self Assessment Checklist that is included in the Step Guide for Improving Theatre Performance.
This will provide a baseline assessment against the standard and will highlight areas of compliance and non compliance from which trusts can target their improvement action plans.

Why patients wait

There are many reasons patients wait. Traditionally, it has been assumed that waiting times are caused by a mismatch of capacity and demand — too many patients and too few resources. We will examine issues around capacity and demand in Chapter 5. But there are other reasons for waits. In this chapter we examine two of the biggest villains in the outpatient system: Patients being seen out of order, and the effects of 'did not attends' (DNAs) on the smooth running of outpatient clinics.

Waiting for an appointment

Imagine that you are sitting in a waiting room on a Monday morning. You are in your local NHS Trust hospital, and you are feeling very pleased with yourself. You knew from your friends, the papers and the TV that there were real problems with the NHS, including long waits for outpatient appointments. Yet you had been to see your GP the previous week, and received an appointment from the hospital a few days later — for later that week! Here you are, only ten days after seeing your GP for what you know is not an urgent problem, and the NHS has been incredibly fast and responsive. You turn to the person sitting next to you.

"Things have certainly improved since I was here last" you say. "I only had to wait ten days to get my appointment this time — maybe all the stuff in the papers about improvements to the NHS is working!"

The person next to you explodes: "TEN DAYS! I have been waiting nearly nine months to get to see this consultant! Why did you get preferential treatment? They better just wait till I get home and get onto my newspaper. Then they'll hear about the efficiency of the NHS!"

You sink back into your seat, subdued. What is going on here?

Two patients, neither an emergency, waiting significantly different times for their appointments. We know that as the GP referrals are sent in to the hospital they are prioritised by the consultant. We know that the appointment clerks make the appointments into the next available slot. Why then is there such a disparity between the two appointment waits?

The answer is simple and repeated thousands of times across the country every day. In this case your companion in the waiting room has probably been 'cancelled' a couple of times. The average wait in this clinic is ten weeks — within the current guidelines for length of wait. When your companion's referral was received, an appointment was made for 10 weeks time. But just before the clinic occurred, the Consultant put in a leave form — and all the patients in the clinic were rescheduled. Unfortunately, all the clinics for the next ten weeks were full (after all, there is a ten week wait, and everyone has their appointment). So a new appointment was made — for another ten week wait.

What about you? Your appointment wasn't cancelled — but surely you would have had to wait at least ten weeks? You were lucky in the cancellation lottery. The day that your letter arrived on the clerk's desk, so did another — from a patient cancelling their appointment for this week. Suddenly there was a free slot — and as your referral was the next to cross the clerk's desk, in you went.

Figure 1 is a graph showing all routine referrals made to one consultant in a typical speciality during one month. Urgent appointments have been excluded. The range of waiting times is from less than one week up to 40 weeks. There is also a cyclical nature to the booking process — as referrals are received, they are processed in batches, affecting the 'next available clinic' time, which may change between batches as adjustments are made to clinics.

FIGURE 1
Variations in Waiting Times

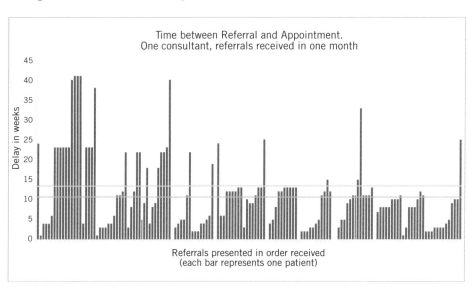

The extreme waits are due to clinic cancellations — these are people who have missed an appointment because either they or the hospital has cancelled, and they have been re-booked. As can be seen from the yellow line marking the 13 week point, more people are seen within 13 weeks than outside (32 over 13 weeks, 119 within). The average wait is 10.8 weeks (the blue line).
The median wait is 9 weeks yet there are 32 patients waiting over 13 weeks.

Waiting in a clinic

Patients being seen out of turn is not the only problem associated with the traditional way of making outpatient appointments. The most common complaint relating to outpatient appointments (after those to do with the time between GP referral and the hospital appointment) is the time people spend in the clinic waiting to see a consultant. Typically a large number of people are waiting at the start of the outpatient clinic; there are always a lot of people in the waiting room, and the clinics run late. Why is this?

Consider a typical outpatient department such as ENT or Ophthalmology, both of which see large numbers of patients in a session. Assume each patient spends 10 minutes with the consultant, or 15 minutes with a registrar.
Over the course of a busy 3 hour clinic, at best 30 patients could be seen by these two doctors. (The actual figures are not important at this stage).

On average 15% of patients do not attend their outpatient appointment. Because there are long waiting times for new referrals, and medical staff are a scarce resource the clinic is overbooked by 15% to account for the DNAs — sensibly, because otherwise, medical staff will be underutilised. This means that there are now 35 patients booked into 30 slots for the afternoon.

What effect does this overbooking have on the smooth running of the clinic? Firstly, although on average there are 15% DNAs, crucially there is no way to know which patients these are. A worst case for the clinic would be for several patients to fail to show for their appointments at the start of the clinic, and all the 'overbooked' patients to be booked at the end. This would mean that the consultant time would still be wasted, but the staff still have to stay late — definitely a lose-lose situation.

What is done, of course, is to overbook the start of the clinic to ensure that there is always a steady supply of patients waiting in the hospital to feed into the consultant. This makes sense from the point of view of protecting a scarce resource, but it leads to overcrowding in waiting rooms, and long waits — because it is a very rare event that the DNAs are all the first patients booked.

Of course, it is a rare event that the DNA rate for a clinic is 15% — the 15% figure is an average, and averages can be dangerous tools.

What is the effect of overbooking by average amounts?
Some clinics, to be sure, will have 15% overbooking and 15% DNAs, and in theory the right number of patients will attend — but NOT at the right times. However, in the worst case from the staff's perspective, some days there will be no DNAs — and they will be faced with an afternoon of full waiting rooms, long waits and finishing late. They will get complaints from patients, and clerks will be blamed for overbooking the clinics.

Surely this will be balanced by the good days — if the average DNA rate is six patients, and sometimes it is none, then surely there are days when twelve patients don't attend the clinic? But the chance that all twelve DNAs will be at the end of the clinic is as rare as the chance that all will be at the beginning. And because these are unannounced non-attendances, even if they were all at the end, you would not know until after the clinic should have concluded. So everyone stays till the end after all. The overrun days cannot be balanced out by days when you finish early — there are no good days to balance the bad.

An example...
This is illustrated by Figure 2 on the next page. The data here come from an ENT consultant, and represent 50 consecutive outpatient clinics. The clinics are all for new patients, and all degrees of urgency are included. The average DNA rate for the 50 clinics used in this example is 14.5%. 19 of the 50 clinics have DNA rates of less than 10%, so with an overbooking rate of 15%, these 19 clinics were overbooked by at least 5% and up to 15%. Another 16 clinics had DNA rates of 10% to 20%, giving slight overbooking or underbooking. And 15 clinics had DNA rates above 20% — which meant that in these cases the clinic was substantially underutilised, because the 'average' overbooking of 15% was not sufficient to compensate for the DNAs in that clinic. In the worst case, half the patients for one particular clinic did not attend!

What are some other consequences?

Patient surveys have shown that waits in clinic are a major concern. Fortunately Trusts no longer ask all patients to come at 2pm for the clinic — but sometimes it still seems that way. Faced with long waits, 'experienced' patients may try to arrive early, to beat the queue, adding to the front-loading problem.

FIGURE 2

Variations in DNA rates

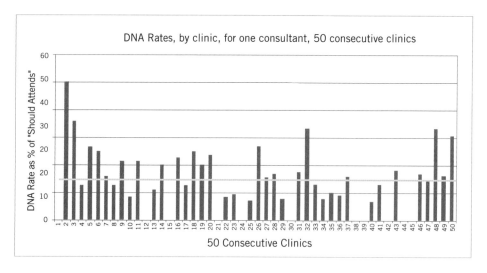

Another problem for patients is often parking. If a patient waits two hours in clinic, their car spends two hours in the car park. If each patient spends only an hour, the number of cars parking will be considerably reduced. The worst parking problems are at the start of clinics — when everyone overbooked and front-loaded arrives at once — along with those patients trying to beat the queue!

But overall, the negative effect of a poorly designed clinic system is most seen in people's attitudes. Patients get disgruntled. Staff get demoralised — consultants are running a clinic where every time they put their heads out into the waiting room they see a sea of faces, all eagerly awaiting their turn — and the pressure of all those people waiting makes them rush patients through. Complaints increase. Parking is a problem so patients are late, adding to the problem.

Clinic flow rates

It is important to understand how an overbooked clinic runs under various situations, and compare these to how a clinic would run if there were no DNAs. To illustrate this, five clinic scenarios are presented as a series of work flow charts, Figures 3a to 3e. Before explaining the figures, it is important to understand the assumptions that they are based on.

The clinic described in these figures is three hours long (2pm until 5pm) with each patient taking approximately 10 minutes with the sole clinician. For each patient, an 'actual time' of between 5 minutes and 15 minutes has been randomly allocated. These average out to 9 minutes, well within the ten minutes the appointment slots allow.

No patient is late or early for their appointment. There are no breaks in the clinic, and under each scenario it is assumed that the clinician does not go faster or slower to cope with the changed workload (which is what normally happens). This scenario presents a simplified view of clinic structure to make the interpretation of the effect (over-booking) easier to observe.

It is also assumed that on average the clinic has a DNA rate of 20%. In a clinic of 18 patients, five extra have been added to compensate for these DNAs. As already discussed, there is no advantage to these additional patients arriving later than a patient who DNAs, so (in figures 3a to 3c) the extra five patients are booked early in the clinic — two at 2pm, and one each at 2:10pm, 2:20pm, and 2:30pm.

On the work-flow graphs, each patient is represented by a horizontal bar. The start of the bar (a black line) represents the patient appointment time. A yellow bar represents a patient wait, and the green portion represents the time that the patient spends with the clinician. If a bar shows only the black portion, the patient at that time was a DNA.

Figure 3a represents a normal clinic. The clinic is 20% overbooked, but five patients DNA, so the number in the clinic is the correct number for the total time available. There are several lengthy waits early in the clinic, but these reduce over time and the clinic finishes a fraction over time, at 5:03pm. The average wait for all patients is only 7 minutes, and the longest wait for a patient is 21 minutes — within patient charter standards.

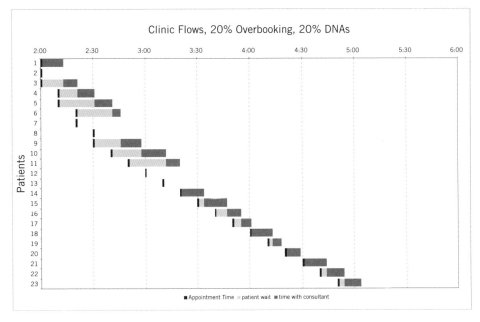

Figure 3b over page represents one of those 'good' days. Although five extra patients are booked, ten do not turn up. As seen in the real case of figure 2, this happens more often than may be thought. Once again the DNAs are randomly allocated through the clinic.

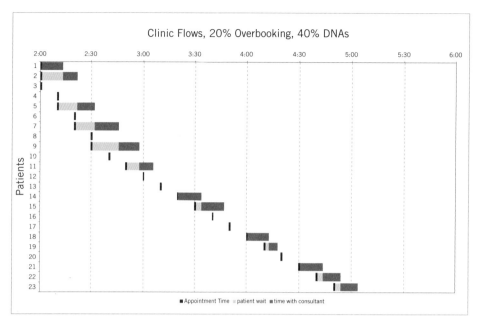

What impact do these five extra DNAs have? The average wait is reduced slightly, from 7 minutes to 5 minutes. The longest wait for a patient is reduced from 21 minutes to 15 minutes. The major effect is that the clinician has 42 minutes unoccupied. The clinic finishes at the same time!

What happens, if instead of five fewer patients, five extra turn up — the example of no DNAs. Figure 3c shows the impact. Average patient waiting goes from 7 minutes to 38, and 17 patients break the charter guidelines of being seen within 30 minutes (two others just scrape in at 29!) The longest wait goes from 21 minutes to 52, but most dramatically, the total time spent by patients in the waiting room goes from 2 hours 16 minutes up to 14 hours 38 minutes!

Crowding also increases. In figure 3a, the maximum number of patients in the waiting room shortly after 2pm was four, but this dropped rapidly. In figure 3c, this remains at six for most of the afternoon. The clinic finishes 43 minutes late.

FIGURE 3C
Clinic Flows,
20% Overbooking and
no DNAs

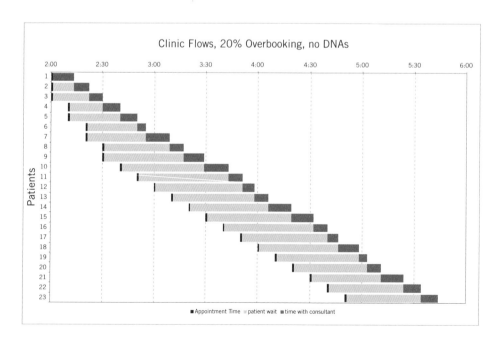

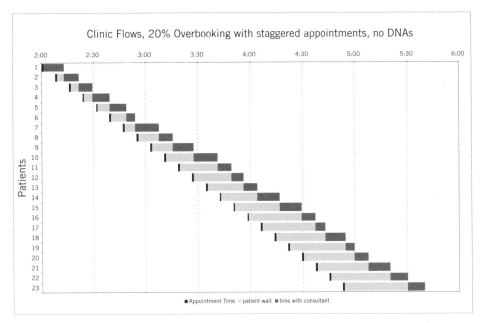

What happens if the clinic is booked with slightly shorter appointment times, staggering the additional patients rather than front loading them? This would spread the increasing waits through the clinic, catching up each time there is a DNA. But as figure 3d shows, when there are no DNAs the waits get steadily longer throughout the afternoon. This scenario also doesn't cope well if there are several DNAs early in the clinic.

The final clinic presented here is figure 3e. This clinic has 18 patients (the optimum amount). It allows 10 minutes per patient as do figures 3a to 3c. However, the average wait is only 3 minutes. The longest wait is 8 minutes, and the total patient waiting time is 54 minutes. No DNAs have been planned for. It has been assumed that every patient will attend, and patients have been booked accordingly. There is no front loading of the clinic to compensate, no shortening of appointment slots to allow for the extra patients.

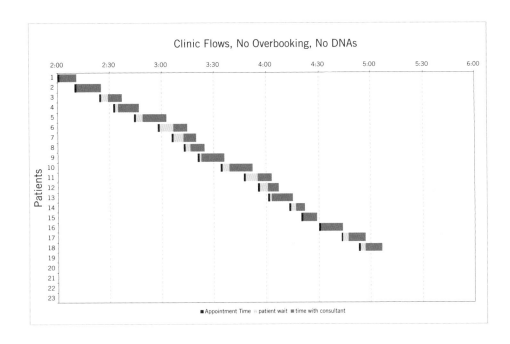

Figure 4 summarises the statistics for these five examples. Probably the most significant fact of these examples is reinforced by graphs 5a and 5b.

These combine the projections for the examples presented plus simulations for all numbers of DNAs between zero and ten. The graphs show the relationship between DNAs and time wasted with increased or decreased numbers of attenders in an overbooked clinic.

FIGURE 4
Summary of the five
clinic scenarios

	Number of patients seen	Total patient/ clinician contact time	Total clinician wait time	Average patient wait	Maximum patient wait	Total patient wait time (all patients)
20% overbooked 20% DNAs	18	2hr 57min	6min	7min	21min	2hr 16min
20% overbooked 40%DNAs	13	2hr 21min	42min	5min	15min	1hr 7min
20% overbooked No DNAs	23	3hr 43min	nil	38min	52min	14hr 28min
20% overbooked staggered, no DNAs	23	3hr 43min	nil	19min	37min	7hr 4min
No overbooking No DNAs	18	2hr 59min	3min	3min	8min	54min

Figure 5a shows that as the number of DNAs goes down, the total amount of wasted patient time increases exponentially. Figure 5b shows that the effect is similar but less pronounced for average and maximum patient waits.

It is clear from these examples that the NHS has historically taken a mistaken approach to the problem of DNAs. It has accepted DNAs as a normal fact of hospital existence, and has worked out strategies to accommodate them.

The approach has dealt with the symptom of the problem, rather than dealing with the root cause. What must be addressed is the reason for DNAs. DNAs must be eliminated from clinics, and booked accordingly. Only then will the NHS get out of the morass that DNAs and strategies to 'fix' them have created.

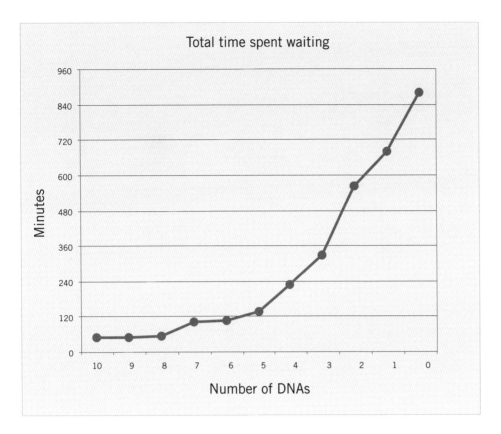

FIGURE 5A
This graph shows the impact of varying DNAs on total time waiting for clinic with 20% overbooking, and 18 patient slots.

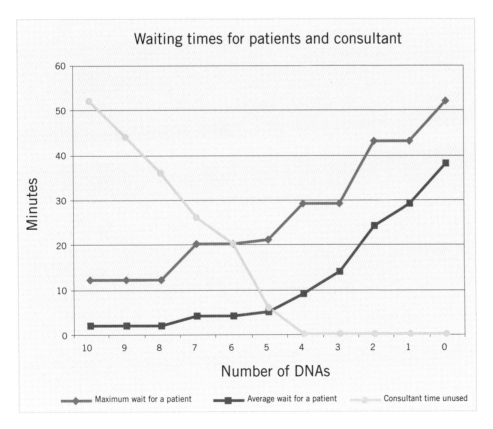

FIGURE 5B
This graph shows the impact of varying DNAs on the average and maximum waits experienced by individual patients, as well as the utilisation of the consultant's time.

Part Two of the Guide looks at the processes around management of waiting lists. Chapter 2 looks at the definitions and processes involved in managing waiting lists; Chapter 3 lays out the process of patient focused booking, the model for making appointments in the NHS in Wales.

Key Points:

■ All patients on the waiting list should be ready for immediate treatment, should the resources be available to treat them tomorrow. Trusts must then manage the waiting list in a way that is fair to the patients, so that waiting times are as short as possible.

■ Waiting lists must be regularly validated using a standard and appropriate process, so that the waiting list reflects a true picture of the number of patients waiting for treatment.

■ Prioritisation must be fair and clinically appropriate, while recognising that increasing levels of prioritisation increases waiting times. Tools such as the Clinically Prioritise and Treat Toolkit can be used to study the effects of prioritisation on waiting times.

■ Primary Targeting Lists, and the use of primary targeting monitoring systems such as the PTLS, will significantly reduce maximum waiting times.

■ Pooling and the use of generic referring will also reduce maximum waiting times.

■ There must be a consistent approach to booking patients for elective treatment in Wales. This approach is called Patient Focused Booking.

■ In Patient Focused Booking, all appointments are made with the involvement of the patient.

■ Appointments are made within time frames that ensure that agreed appointments will occur; this means that firm appointment dates and times are only agreed up to six weeks into the future. Appointments further into the future are 'partially' booked.

■ The patient focused booking process applies to all elective contacts with the hospital; outpatients (new and return appointments) elective surgery, and diagnostic and therapy appointments.

All elective admissions are pre-assessed in an outpatient setting as part of this process.

Managing waiting lists

2

Sometimes it seems that the NHS is primarily about waiting lists. Public perception focuses on waiting lists. Waiting lists provide media headlines. For those working within the NHS, it seems that too often the real work of staff is lost in a concern for waiting times and targets.

There is some truth to this position. Waiting times are an easy target for the media. Waiting times are measurable, where so much else in the NHS is not. Many waiting times are long. It is easy to set targets for waiting times reductions.

There is one fundamental truth behind this rhetoric.
Many waiting times are too long.

What can be done to reduce waiting times? Chapter 2 deals with basic waiting list management: definitions, validation, prioritisation and the use of primary targeting lists. It also includes a chapter on the improvement tool 'Clinically Prioritise and Treat' used by the *Implementing the Guide to Good Practice Programme*, and the calculation and use of PTL rates and scores, used for performance management in the NHS in Wales from April 2005.

Understanding the definitions
The Welsh Assembly Government uses a formalised structure to monitor waiting times across Wales. The definitions used in this process are included in 2.2.

Validation
Validation of waiting lists must be routine. 2.3 covers the principles of validation and provides sample scripts and letters.

Clinical prioritisation
Clinical prioritisation is often suggested as a key factor in managing waiting lists, 2.4 looks at what levels of prioritisation are appropriate.

Use of the CPaT toolkit
The Clinically Prioritise and treat Toolkit was developed by the Modernisation Agency as a tool to help discussions between clinicians and managers about good waiting list practice. 2.5 describes the toolkit and its application.

Primary targeting lists

Primary targeting lists involve the ordered treatment of patients by referral date, and 2.6 covers how primary targeting reduces waiting times for inpatients and outpatients.

PTL Rates and scores

2.7 covers measurement of PTL implementation, an important tool in performance management which is now integral to the performance management process in Wales

There are waiting lists in the NHS because lists are not managed well. This situation must change. The techniques outlined in this chapter are fundamental, and must be adopted in the management of all waiting lists, be they inpatient, daycase, outpatient or for diagnostic tests.

CONWY & DENBIGHSHIRE NHS TRUST
Pooled outpatient lists

The development of a pooled outpatient waiting list in the Ophthalmic Directorate ensures that patients of the same clinical priority are seen in chronological order. This practice enables patients on the waiting list to be placed within a single queue rather than multiple waiting queues and ensures equity of access.

Objectives:

- *Equalise waiting times for patients' first appointments*
- *Assist in the modernisation of patient access to hospital services*
- *Improve the service to patients thus improve patient satisfaction*

Booking procedure:

1. *Senior Medical Officer to indicate urgency — routine or specify when patient to be seen.*
2. *Indicate — diagnosis, procedure.*
3. *Patient entered on outpatient waiting list entry screen and acknowledgement letter sent. No consultant selected at this stage.*
4. *Patient selected in order of wait.*
5. *Consultant selected and entered on PAS.*
6. *Second letter sent to patient requesting they contact the appointment clerk to arrange their appointment.*
7. *Patient contact made regarding appointment. Consultant and location can be altered at patient's request at this stage.*

This process came into practice September 2003 and is managed referencing specific clinical requirements within the specialty of ophthalmology, with subspecialties such as vitreo-retinal surgery dealt with by the identified consultant specialist. As the majority of ophthalmic referrals are suitable for the pool this will make a significant difference to the equity and efficiency of ophthalmic patient services at the point of referral.

Understanding the definitions

This chapter contains definitions of specific terms used through this manual. It also contains the Welsh Assembly Government guidance on how patients should be managed for waiting list measurement reasons. These definitions are updated from previous data definitions, and were confirmed in Welsh Health Circulars WHC (2004) 40 and 41, and Change Control Notices 01/2004(W) and 02/2004(W), all issued on 7th June 2004.

Clinical Referral Date (CRD)

The Clinical Referral Date (CRD) is the clinically significant date marking the start of a period of waiting either for an initial outpatient consultation or for an episode of treatment such as elective surgery. The CRD is used to order pick lists used for booking patients, and it does not change under any circumstance. It is not used to calculate performance waiting time statistics.

Outpatients

The Clinical Referral Date (CRD) is the date that the referral of an outpatient appointment is received in the Trust. All referrals should be date stamped on opening, and entered onto the PAS with the date stamped date as the CRD. The CRD is used to order the lists for partial booking pick lists.

Inpatient and Day case events

The Clinical Referral Date (CRD) or the decision to admit (DTA) date is the date that a decision was made by a clinician within the Trust (or a GP outside the Trust in cases of direct access referrals) to list the patient for treatment. The CRD or DTA date is used to order the waiting list for selection of patients for surgery.

Waiting List Date (WLD)

The waiting list entry date (WLD) is initially set as the same date as the Clinical Referral Date (CRD). The WLD is used to calculate waiting times for the purposes of measuring Trust performance against Welsh Assembly Government performance targets. It is not used to order out-patient waiting lists for partial booking or to order in-patient or day case lists for selection of patients for surgery.

There are a number of situations where the WLD may be changed. These include rescheduling an appointment at the patient's request, reinstatement to a waiting list following removal, or where a patient has chosen to remain with a consultant when offered an earlier appointment with a different consultant. The circumstances where the WLD may be changed are covered in the various definitions in this section.

The CRD or DTA date are never changed. The WLD may be changed.

GOOD PRACTICE POINT

Waiting Lists

A patient should only be placed on a waiting list when all preconditions for treatment have been met. As a test, no patient should be active on a surgical waiting list unless the procedure could be performed tomorrow if the appropriate resources were available.

Did Not Phone (DNP)

Any patient who does not phone in response to a partial booking letter or a validation letter may, once certain preconditions have been met, be removed from the waiting list with the reason for removal being 'DNP'.

Treatment of DNPs

Under partial booking a DNP should be recorded only where the required number of reminder letters have been sent, and the required time for a response has lapsed. In most cases this will mean an initial letter and a reminder letter have been sent (two weeks apart) and a further two weeks after the second letter has elapsed.

A DNP should be removed from the waiting list and suitable notification made.

Minimum Standard

The patient's referring GP or GDP should be notified that the patient has failed to phone and has therefore been removed from the waiting list. Instructions should be included on how the patient can be returned to the waiting list (see sample letter on page 79). Instructions should also be included on what to do if the patient has a serious condition that requires urgent attention.

Good Practice

The patient should be notified that they have been removed from the waiting list because they have failed to respond to two requests to contact the Trust. Information should be included that tells the patient how to get re-referred if they now or subsequently have problems (see page 79).

Did Not Attend (DNA)

A Did Not Attend (DNA) is recorded where a patient does not attend any appointment or admission within the Trust without notifying the Trust.

Treatment of DNAs

Any patient who fails to attend their appointment or admission should be removed from the appropriate waiting list and suitable notifications made.

Minimum Standard

The patient's referring GP or GDP should be notified that the patient has failed to attend their appointment or admission and has therefore been removed from the waiting list. Instructions should be included on how the patient can be returned to the waiting list. Instructions should also be included on what to do if the patient has a serious condition that requires urgent attention. Where the appointment was for a follow-up outpatient appointment or for an admission event, the person requesting the appointment or admission (eg the consultant in the previous outpatient clinic) should also be notified.

Good Practice

The patient should be notified that they have been removed from the waiting list because they have failed to attend their clinic or admission event. Information should be included that tells the patient how to get re-referred if they subsequently have problems.

Could Not Attend (CNA)

A Could Not Attend (CNA) is recorded where a patient notifies the Trust that they will not be able to attend an appointment or admission event, up to the end of the day of their appointment or admission.

Treatment of CNAs

First CNA

Any patient who contacts the Trust to notify it that they will be unable attend an outpatient appointment or admission event should have another appointment or event arranged at the time of the notification. If the patient notifies by phone, the new appointment should be made then. If the patient notifies by letter or email, an immediate response should be sent asking the patient to contact the Trust by phone to arrange a new appointment.

At the time of contact, the Waiting List entry Date (WLD) should be reset to the date of the contact with the patient. In most cases this will be the current date.

Second CNA

When a patient contacts the Trust to cancel a second appointment the Trust may treat the cancellation as a DNA and not make an appointment. In this case, the communication standards for a DNA must be followed.

Minimum Standard

The patient's referring GP or GDP should be notified that the patient has cancelled two consecutive appointments or admissions and has therefore been removed from the waiting list. Instructions should be included on how the patient can be returned to the waiting list. Instructions should also be included on what to do if the patient has a serious condition that requires urgent attention. Where the appointment was for a follow-up outpatient appointment or for an admission event, the person requesting the appointment or admission (eg the consultant in the previous outpatient clinic) should also be notified.

Good Practice

The patient should be notified that they have been removed from the waiting list because they have cancelled two consecutive outpatient clinic appointments or admission events. Information should be included that tells the patient how to get re-referred if they now or subsequently have problems.

Reinstatement to the waiting list

Reinstatement to the waiting list can be made by a reasonable request from the patient, or by an authorised Trust employee or the patient's GP or GDP. The patient will be reinstated on the waiting list with their Waiting List Date (WLD) set to the date of the request for reinstatement. No reinstatement to a waiting list should take place more than three months from the date of removal. In these cases the patient will require a new GP referral.

Reinstatement will follow removal for one of a number of reasons. Patients may be removed because they were a DNA or DNP, because they were a multiple CNA, or because they failed to respond to validation or responded that they wished to be removed from the list. Reinstatement may be requested in all cases by the patient, Trust employee (usually a clinician) or the patient's referring GP or GDP.

A reasonable request from the patient for reinstatement could be either clinical (because a condition has recurred or got worse since removal) or social (the patient may have been away from home when the validation letter or partial booking letter was received, and will ask for reinstatement on their return). In all cases the patient will be returned to the waiting list with their Waiting List Date (WLD) set to the date of the request for reinstatement.

Reinstatement by Trust staff or the patient's GP will usually be for clinical reasons. The GP will ask that the patient be reinstated because their condition has not improved and the original reasons for referral still exist. The Consultant will ask for reinstatement to the waiting list or follow-up outpatient clinic because they believe that the patient continues to need treatment within the Trust.

In all such cases, indication should be sought from the clinician as to what steps will be taken to ensure the patient's attendance at subsequent appointments. While a patient may be reinstated, simple reinstatement to a waiting list or making of a further appointment does not meet the obligation of the clinician to see the patient where there is a clinical need for the reinstatement.

Where the reinstatement has been requested by a consultant, the consultant should contact the patient's GP to determine whether reinstatement is the best option, and to enlist the assistance of the GP in ensuring the patient's attendance at subsequent appointments. Where the reinstatement is at the GP's request, the GP should first contact the patient to find out why the patient did not attend, and to ensure that the patient will attend subsequently.

Where a request is made to reinstate a patient to a waiting list who has been removed from a waiting list or clinic because of two or more non-attendances or non-responses, the request for reinstatement should be made through the clinical head of the service involved. It must be emphasised that simple reinstatement or making a new appointment is not treatment of the patient, and if the patient requires treatment, avenues must be followed that will lead to the attendance of the patient, not simple reinstatement.

Change of care provider or treatment location

Trusts may ask patients whether they are prepared to be seen by a different care provider or at a different location than was originally intended. In all cases, the patient may exercise their right of choice and choose to remain with the original clinician or location.

In order to reduce overall waiting times, Trusts may pool waiting lists. This will involve moving patients from the care of one health professional to another, or from one location to another. A patient may be moved to a consultant of equivalent sub-specialisation who has a shorter waiting list; to a non-consultant clinic (such as a GPSI or advanced practice physiotherapist), or to a clinic held by the same consultant at a different location. All pooling after an initial offer of information must be subject to the agreement of the patient.

This means that where the Trust has notified a patient that they are on the outpatient waiting list of a particular consultant, they must contact the patient in person or by letter before pooling the referral. Similarly, if a patient has seen a specific consultant in clinic and been placed on that consultant's inpatient waiting list, the consent of the patient must be granted to transfer them to another consultant's inpatient list.

Where pooling is policy and normal practice for a service, or where referrals will be routinely seen by a non-consultant as part of an alternative pathway of care, individual consent does not need to be sought from the patient. In this case it is important that the policy and the current practices are made clear to all GPs who may refer into the Trust and to all staff within the Trust, so that patients are given clear information about pooling when they are referred. Confirmation of the receipt of referral should also include a statement about the pooling policies of the Trust (see letter on page 78).

If the patient exercises their right to remain with an original consultant or clinic location their consultant or clinic will not be changed, however the Waiting List Date (WLD) will be reset to the date of the decision. This means that the patient will no longer show as a long wait on the original list. This does not affect their position on the waiting list however. They will remain in their existing position on the list for the purpose of generating the Primary Targeting List (PTL), as the PTL sort is done on the basis of the original Clinical Referral Date (CRD) not the WLD.

When a patient exercises their right to remain with an original consultant or clinic location, they must be advised at the time of choice that the decision may mean that their wait will be longer than if they accept the change. They should also be advised that they will no longer fall within the waiting times targets set by the Welsh Assembly Government. Some sample wording can be found in the letter on page 78.

In some Trusts, routine validation of long wait patients includes an offer to transfer care to an alternative consultant or care provider. In some cases the validation may offer treatment at an alternative facility. In these cases, the validation process should be seen as part of the pooling process. Where patients decline to be pooled, their WLD should be reset to the date of the validation letter. In these cases the consequences of declining the offer of pooling must be clearly spelt out in the validation letter.

This process is covered in the chapter on pooling on page 55 and a sample validation letter can be found on page 33.

Sometimes patients are referred to the wrong consultant or speciality, or a second opinion is sought. Referrals to the incorrect consultant, which are then forwarded to a *different consultant within the same speciality*, should be treated as follow-up appointments. Transfers to a different Trust (tertiary referrals) or to a different speciality in the same Trust, should be treated as a new referral. Transfers from an alternative care provider (such as a physiotherapy triage clinic) should be treated as a follow-up appointment.

Suspending patients

Patients may be suspended on both inpatient and outpatient waiting lists. The rules for suspension are the same for all cases. Patients can only be suspended for a period of up to six months, with the exception of suspensions for pregnancy. Where the patient is not available for treatment at the end of six months they will be removed from the waiting list.

Patients can be suspended for two categories; either because they are medically unfit for surgery (medical suspensions) or because they have non-medical reasons why they are unavailable for surgery or the appointment (social reasons).

A patient cannot be re-suspended for the same reason after the six month period is up. A patient may be re-suspended for a period for a different reason. For example, a patient may be suspended for social reasons for a period of three months and then found to be unfit for surgery at pre-assessment. They could be suspended for a further six months to stabilise their medical condition.

Medical suspensions
Patients are suspended for medical reasons when they are temporarily unfit to undergo the procedure for which they are waiting. One example of this would be when a patient is seen in a preoperative assessment clinic and found to be unfit for surgery.

Patients suspended for medical reasons can only be suspended for a maximum period of six months. There must be robust mechanisms in place to deal with the reason for the suspension. In cases where the patient is unfit for surgery a plan must be in place to ensure that when the suspension period ends, the patient will be fit.

For example, if when a patient is pre-assessed they are found to have a number of medical conditions that would exclude them from surgery due to unfitness, this patient cannot be suspended for a period of six months for one of the medical conditions and then re-suspended for an additional six months for another of the pre-existing medical conditions that were detected at the original point of suspension. All the patient's medical conditions detected at the original point of suspension should be managed within the six months period. If they are not resolved at the end of the six months period, this patient should be removed from the waiting list. However, if a patient is found to have developed another medical condition, the patient can be re-suspended for an additional six months.

Where the responsibility falls on the patient's GP to ensure that their medical reason for suspension is dealt with, the Trust must have in place processes to ensure that the GP is notified of;

- the suspension and the time limit on the suspension;
- the clinical actions that need to be taken to ensure that the patient is fit for surgery;
- the consequences of the suspension period ending while the patient is still unfit.

If the patient is not fit by the end of the six months, they will be removed from the waiting list and not placed back on the list until they are fit for surgery.

In one case the maximum period of six months can be extended. In the case of pregnancy, a patient may be suspended for a period of longer than six months, provided that an end date is recorded.

Where a patient is admitted for surgery which is subsequently cancelled because the patient has an underlying medical problem, the patient is managed as a suspension for medical reasons.

Social suspensions

Patients are suspended for social reasons when they are unavailable for their appointment or admission for reasons other than a medical condition.
One example may be a patient going overseas for a period, or a student may be studying away from home. A patient may also be a social suspension if they are unavailable because they are caring for a relative.

When the patient notifies the Trust that they are unavailable for an appointment or admission for social reasons, the end point of the suspension will be the point at which the patient becomes available for treatment.

Where a patient is suspended for social reasons, the maximum period of suspension will not be longer than six months.

The patient's suspension from the waiting list should end automatically at either the negotiated date or after six months, whichever is sooner.

Patients should not be suspended for social reasons for a total of more than six months, i.e. if a patient is suspended for 3 months because they are on holiday, they can only be suspended for social reasons for a further maximum of 3 months.

Administrative processes after suspension

It is unlikely that a patient will be able to have their admission or their appointment the day that their suspension ends. Once a suspension ends, the patient will feed back into the normal administrative process described elsewhere in this document. This means that there will be a period of up to six weeks from the time the patient is available for an appointment and the appointment occurring. Where patients are close to maximum waiting times at the point of suspension, this may mean that the normal partial booking approach will lead to waiting list breaches.

For this reason it is recommended that Trusts differentiate between when a patient is available to make an appointment and when the patient is available for the appointment. Patients will be available for an appointment or admission six weeks subsequent to being available to make the appointment. This six weeks should be built into the suspension period, and the patient contact process should start six weeks before the end of the suspension.

Trusts cannot insert a six week booking window on the end of a maximum six months suspension period.

Two examples should make this clear. Patient A is going overseas, and will not be available to make an appointment until their return. If they are going overseas for ten weeks, they will not be available to make an appointment until week eleven. Because partial booking covers a window of up to six weeks, the patient may not attend an appointment until week sixteen. The suspension should therefore be set to 16 weeks, not ten. They should receive the partial booking 'phone in' letter in week ten, six weeks before the end of the suspension period.

Patient B is booked for surgical pre-assessment, but at the pre-assessment clinic they are determined to have an underlying medical problem that can be stabilised in three months (13 weeks). A letter is written to the GP explaining the course of treatment required over the three months, and the patient is suspended. Patient B will be available for pre-assessment in 13 weeks. They are not out of contact so before the end of the 13 weeks the booking process can recommence. Because there is a delay of up to six weeks but typically four weeks between letter and pre-assessment appointment, and because there is no point to bringing the patient to pre-assessment before 13 weeks, the 'phone in' letter should be generated in week nine. The suspension should exceed the phone in date by six weeks, so the suspension should be set to 15 weeks (not 13) and the phone-in letter generated six weeks before the end of the suspension period.

When calculating the WLD, periods of suspension for either medical or social reasons should not be included. This means that when a patient is placed back on the active waiting list, the WLD should be changed to reflect the period of suspension. For example, if the WLD was 12 October 2004 and the patient was suspended for two months, the WLD would become 12 December 2004.

Deferments where a patient has not complied with instructions
In some cases surgery or investigative procedures require that the patient undergo a period of preparation at home prior to admission or attendance. One example would be the requirement to fast before surgery; another would be bowel preparation before colonoscopy or barium enema. Sometimes patients attend their admission or appointment without having completed the required preparation, and the procedure cannot be undertaken.

In these cases the patient should be treated as a CNA. Time must be taken to explain to the patient why the procedure cannot be undertaken, and the new date for the procedure should be negotiated with the patient. It is also important that the preparation instructions are discussed fully with the patient or their carer so that the situation does not recur. The WLD will be reset to the current date as part of the CNA process, and multiple noncompliance would also fall within the CNA process.

Where a particular procedure has a high degree of noncompliance it is important to review the literature and instructions sent to the patient to determine if they are clear. Alternative methods of conveying the required information to the patient should be investigated.

Reasonable offer

An essential part of these definitions is that any offer to the patient is reasonable. Where patients are being removed for DNA or CNA the appointment must have been for a reasonable offer of appointment or admission as defined below.

Patients cannot be removed for DNA or CNA where a reasonable offer did not exist.

Where a patient does not agree to an offer defined below as reasonable, they may, at the discretion of the Trust, be recorded as a CNA. However, a suitable appointment should still be agreed. The recording as a CNA purely affects the recording of the waiting time on the Trust performance monitoring systems.

Normal outpatient appointment

A normal outpatient appointment may be an appointment of any clinical priority. A reasonable offer must include the following factors:

■ The patient must have been involved in agreeing to the appointment date and time, either by phone or in person;
■ The patient must have been offered a choice of at least three possible dates and times, one of which must be at least four weeks into the future.
■ The appointment will normally be at a Trust site, with Trust clinical staff. If the appointment is offered at a site outside the boundaries of the Trust, transport must be offered from a Trust facility. If non-Trust staff will be used, the patient must be advised at the time of the booking being made, and the patient advised that if they choose to decline the appointment, their waiting time may increase.

Outpatient appointment under two weeks

The short time frame involved with organising two week waits usually precludes the possibility of writing to the patient and asking them to phone the Appointment Centre.

In this case, the patient must still be involved in the appointment process. It may be necessary to phone the patient, the appointment may be arranged while the patient is at the GP surgery, or the GP may hand the patient a form asking them to phone the Appointment Centre.

The patient must be offered a choice of two date/times for the appointment, at least one of which must be more than 24 hours into the future.

Diagnostic procedure

Diagnostic Procedures should work to the same definitions of reasonable as outpatients.

Therapeutic outpatient appointment

Therapeutic Services should work to the same definitions of reasonable as outpatients.

The inpatient and day case admission process should be treated as a two stage process.

Preoperative Assessment

The preoperative assessment may be undertaken by phone or in person. Good practice is for on-site preoperative assessment, so that consent may be taken during the assessment appointment.

If the assessment is done by phone, the patient should be sent a letter asking them to phone the clinic at one of a specific set of dates and times. There should be at least four date/time combinations, and one should be at least four weeks into the future.

If an on-site clinic is held, the same parameters apply as for an ordinary outpatient appointment.

Surgical admission

The date and time for admission should be agreed while the patient is present at the preoperative assessment appointment. The patient should be given a choice of two admission dates within the six weeks following the assessment.

Validation

Over time, waiting lists become out of date. Patients may require treatment when they are first added to the list, but circumstances may change. They may choose to have treatment at another location (either in the NHS or in private practice). They may move to another town. Their condition may improve so that treatment is not required. They may die. Systems must be in place to ensure that these patients are removed from the waiting list.

What does validation achieve?

Validation ensures that figures of patient numbers waiting are accurate. Where waiting lists are high, Trust performance may appear to be worse than it actually is if waiting lists contain high numbers of people who are not actually waiting for treatment. This may affect the commissioning process, as the perception may be that there is a more significant volume to be treated.

It may affect information given to patients, who will think that they may have a longer wait than is actually the case. It may also lead to wasted clinical time if clinics are booked through traditional systems and patients not requiring to be seen are given appointments for treatment.

Patient focused booking and self-validation

Patient focused booking (partial booking) is often referred to as self validating. This is because no action is taken by the Trust to allocate resources to the patient's care until the patient has contacted the appointment centre and confirmed that they will be attending, and a date for treatment is agreed. For this reason, it is assumed that validation is not necessary once patient focussed booking is in place.

This is only true when the maximum waiting times for treatment are short. While patient focussed booking will validate patients before they are called for treatment, it does not do so until the patient reaches the top of the waiting list. Where waiting times are long, waiting lists will remain inflated if the lists are not validated at interim stages.

Frequency of validation

There is a need to balance the gains from validation against the time and cost of undertaking it. More importantly, there are issues to do with the reaction of patients and their GPs to the validation process. The NLIAH recommends six monthly validation to achieve this balance.

GOOD PRACTICE POINT

Validation

On all waiting lists, validation should be undertaken at the point the patient is placed on the list, then at six months, and again at 12 months. In the exceptional circumstance where a patient waits over 12 months, validation should be repeated at 18 months and then at six monthly intervals.

Cost of validation

Validation can be done by mail or by telephone. Either includes a cost. Mail validation will have costs associated with letter production and postage, phone validation will have costs associated with phone charges, but by far the most significant cost in both cases will be for the staff time involved. It is vital to balance the benefits of validation against this use of resource. It is also important, where validation is done, to get the best value for the money spent.

Mail validation letters must be clear and targeted at identifying those patients who have either had their surgery, or whose condition has improved so that surgery is no longer necessary. Simple requests as to whether the patient wishes to remain on the waiting list are inadequate.

Validation letters must be clear and unambiguous. The validation process involves removal of patients from the waiting list if they do not respond to the validation letter, and this must be made clear to the patient. Removal of non-responding patients must be completed. Where patients are not removed from the list despite non-response, they should be told why their name has been reinstated.

Telephone validation should be scripted. Questions should be phrased such that the desired information is elicited; asking a patient whether they wish to remain on the waiting list will result in fewer removals than questions that ask if the patient is still having clinical problems. It is also important to make clear to the patient that there are mechanisms for getting back on the list if their condition worsens within a specific time period.

Sample phone scripts and letters can be found on page 33.

Patient responses to validation

Validation can be an imposition on patients, and too frequent validation will lead to patient complaints. If the only communication that a patient receives from a Trust is a three monthly letter asking whether they wish to remain on the waiting list, it is easy to see why they may become annoyed. The more frequent the validation and the longer the list, the more patient perception of the process will become a problem.

Some early documents from Innovations in Care recommended three monthly validation. Frequent validation will have diminishing returns, with fewer removals each time the validation is performed.

Most removals come from the first validation. There are a number of reasons for this; patients are removed from a list because they have had surgery elsewhere, or because their condition has changed. For a number of less serious problems, improvement is more likely to be in the first six months. There will be a high removal rate for this validation.

The NLIAH recommends that subsequent validation be done at intervals of six months. There is no need to do validation close to the appointment time, so where waiting times are 12 months a second validation would be unnecessary. Similarly, where the speciality is working to an 18 month target, the 18 month validation would not be required as the partial booking process will satisfy the validation requirements.

There are two ways in which validation can be timed — in bulk or continually. The trust may decide to do bulk validation at six monthly intervals — all ENT validation in February and August for example. This approach has disadvantages. The validation workload is intensive, and if done episodically, will lead to significant peaks in workload. Additionally, the purpose of validation is to link it to the patient process, and if a speciality undertakes six monthly validation exercises, patients will be validated at less than six months on the list, or may wait up to 11 months before being validated. For this reason, where bulk validation is the only option, it needs to be done more frequently, although each patient should receive validation letters only six monthly.

Continual validation can be generated by the PAS. Procedures in the PAS should automatically generate validation letters at the point where the wait hits six and 12 months. The advantage of this is that there are small numbers of letters generated every week, rather than very large numbers every few months, and the validation process can be handled as part of the ongoing work of the department rather than as an infrequent additional task.

Continual validation also ensures that small numbers of patients are removed each week, rather than large numbers at the end of a longer period. Infrequent 'bulk' validation will lead to artificial peaks and drops in patient waiting list numbers, where continual validation will not.

The validation process at referral
Validation of patient data at referral is not normally thought of as validation, and is often overlooked. On referral, and at each subsequent stage of the administrative process, all patient details must be verified. This must happen on referral, at each outpatient appointment, when the patient is placed on a waiting list, at the pre-operative assessment and at admission. If the details differ from the PAS, the PAS must be updated!

Placing the patient on the outpatient waiting list
GPs re-refer patients to the same Trust, and to different consultants within the Trust. When a new referral is received, the first step should be to see if that patient is already waiting for an appointment, or is currently on the inpatient waiting list for that speciality. If so, the GP should be contacted to determine why the patient has been re-referred.

As part of the patient focused booking process, it is necessary to contact patients by mail and sometimes by phone. It is vital that up to date information is stored on the PAS to allow that contact to happen. On receipt of a referral from a GP, the referral must be checked by clerical staff to ensure that all necessary information is included. Where it is not, the GP must be contacted and the full demographic information requested. Patients must not be added to waiting lists with incomplete demographics.

Where a referral is incomplete and *not* flagged by the GP as urgent, it should be recorded as received but returned to the GP practice with a form requesting the remaining information. The form should note that the referral cannot be received or actioned without complete demographic information. Where the referral is flagged as urgent it should be processed as complete but the GP practice should be contacted by phone for the remaining information.

Demographic information received at referral may go out of date when the waiting times are long. The partial booking acknowledgement letter must include a request that the patient phone the Trust Appointment Centre if any demographic details change while the patient is on the waiting list. This will ensure that records are kept up to date. A sample letter is found on page 78.

Placing the patient on the elective waiting list

When a patient is listed for a diagnostic procedure or surgery, it is imperative to check the demographic details at that point. The person placing the patient on the list should confirm the demographic details with the patient present, and ensure that inaccuracies are corrected.

As with the outpatient acknowledgement letter, the letter confirming placement on a diagnostic or treatment waiting list should include a request to contact the Trust appointment centre if any demographic information changes.

Administrative validation

Administrative validation is undertaken by management and clerical staff, and is primarily designed to determine whether the patient details are correct, and whether the patient wishes to remain on the waiting list.

Administrative validation is undertaken by mail or by phone and has already been covered. Sample letters and scripts will be found on page 33.

Clinical validation

Clinical validation is a more complex, and more time consuming, process. The purpose of clinical validation is to determine whether the patient's clinical condition has changed in any way that may lead to their removal from the waiting list.

Clinical validation can be undertaken by GPs or by Trust staff. In the case of outpatient referral waiting lists, it is by default the GP who will need to undertake the validation. The Trust may supply the practice or the LHB with practice based lists of patients waiting for an outpatient appointment, and the medical records of those patients are reviewed to ensure that the patient still requires the appointment. Although the review process is undertaken in primary care, any contact to the patient advising them that their status has changed should be undertaken by the Trust, which has requested the validation.

In the case of validation of diagnostic or treatment lists, the clinical validation can be performed in the Trust, or in primary care, or both.

Trust based validation can be either a review of the notes, or a clinical reassessment of the patient. Notes review will have limited value, as it is unlikely that any information will be included in the record that will not have already been acted upon. However there can be considerable value to bringing patients into the Trust for reassessment if they have not been seen for some time.

These review appointments can be with consultant staff, but may also be by appropriately trained Allied Health Professionals, such as physiotherapists or nurses working to predetermined protocols.

KEY VALIDATION POINTS

- *Check that a patient is not already on a waiting list before adding them.*
- *Check the patient details at every stage of the administrative process.*
- *Validate continually, rather than in batches.*
- *Balance the advantages against the cost of validation when determining the frequency of validation.*
- *Validation should be undertaken on a six monthly basis as a minimum.*
- *Carefully check wording of validation letters, and telephone scripts.*
- *Undertake clinical validation where possible, in addition to administrative validation.*

GP based review of treatment waiting lists will also identify those patients whose condition has rendered them unfit for surgery. The GP may be treating the patient for an unrelated problem, which has arisen since initial referral, and would now mean that treatment is not possible. GP validation would normally be done by notes review, although in the case of patients who have not been seen for some time in primary care, it may be necessary to see the patient.

FIGURE 6
Validation letters and scripts

VALIDATION PHONE SCRIPT

The following questions should be asked, using the wording provided:

Good morning / afternoon / evening.

My name is ... and I work for the ... NHS Trust.

I am phoning you about your referral to see Dr... in the ... Department.

Are you still having the problem that your GP referred you to Dr... with?

If yes:

Do you still require an appointment to see Dr...

If no:

In that case, is there any reason why you need to remain on the waiting list for Dr...?

If removed:

You can be asked to be put back on the waiting list if your condition gets worse in the next three months. If that happens, please phone 012 345 6789 or contact your GP.

Can you please confirm that the following contact details are correct **(check demographics)**

Do you have any questions about your referral or anything else I can help you with?

Thank you for allowing me the time to ask you these questions.

VALIDATION LETTER
for inpatient, outpatient or day case surgery

Dear ...,

You have been waiting for an appointment to see Dr... since ...date.... You have not been overlooked and your appointment is still pending.

Sometimes patients change address or decide that they no longer want to see the Consultant and forget to let us know. So that we are sure that we have the correct details we write to patients about every six months to check.

We may be able to offer shorter waiting times with a different consultant. If you do not wish to be offered a shorter waiting time with a different consultant, please indicate this on the form.

To keep our records up to date please complete the form overleaf and return it to me in the enclosed reply-paid envelope.

If you need any further help please do not hesitate to contact me between 9am and 5pm Monday to Friday on ...

Yours sincerely

Please tick whichever applies to you:

☐ I still want an appointment

☐ I have an appointment and I am going to keep it

☐ I have had my appointment elsewhere so I no longer need an appointment

☐ I no longer want an appointment in this consultant's clinic

☐ I wish to remain with the current consultant, even if this means I may wait longer for my appointment

If you no longer want the appointment please discuss this with your GP

If you have any comments to make about your choices, please write them below

Has your address or phone changed from those at the top of this page?

If they have please write the new one below. Please let us have any home, work and mobile phone numbers.

Address ...

telephone: home... work ... mobile ...

FIGURE 7

Information leaflet
produced by the Conwy
and Denbighshire NHS
Trust, sent out with all
validation letters

CONWY AND DENBIGHSHIRE NHS TRUST

Validation Information Leaflet produced by the Data Quality Team

These are the answers to some of the questions patients regularly ask when they receive their first letter from us.

Why are you sending me these letters?

■ *We need to make sure our records are kept up to date so it is essential that when you receive one of these letters you return it fully completed. It is important to remember that if you change your mind about coming to clinic or having your procedure, you must let us know straight away. Your appointment could be given to someone else. If you don't keep your appointment for any reason it means that somebody else has to wait a little bit longer for their appointment.*

How long will I have to wait for a date?

■ *This depends on which Consultant and Speciality you are waiting to see and the reason you are waiting. We are doing everything we can to keep your waiting time as short as possible.*

■ *The Data Quality Team can give you an up to date waiting time. If they are unable to help you they will put you in touch with somebody who can.*

What do I do if I want the date of my appointment to be deferred?

■ *Some patients ask to be deferred because they are pregnant, working away from home, or not ready for a visit to hospital. You will still be sent an administration letter. This is because you may change your mind about your appointment/ procedure or may change your address. However we are still aware that you wish to be deferred and that you still require an appointment. You will not be forgotten.*

What happens if the hospital cancels my appointment?

■ *If your appointment is cancelled by the hospital, you will still receive an administration letter. This is because you are still on the waiting list but just waiting for an alternative date.*

■ *Only if you, your GP or the Consultant decide, will your name be removed from the waiting list. If you do not let us know you have been treated elsewhere we will still send you these letters.*

Do I need to let the hospital know if I change address?

■ *It is important for you to let us know as quickly as possible if you are moving to a new address. If we are not able to contact you, you could be removed from the waiting list.*

■ *You also need to tell your GP your new address.*

Clinical prioritisation

Traditionally patients on waiting lists have been prioritised according to a simple system: they are either 'Urgent', 'Soon' or 'Routine'. These categories are used for both inpatient waiting lists and for newly referred patients awaiting an outpatient appointment. Little thought is given to definitions for these terms, yet they have been fundamental to the development of waiting lists.

The 'traditional definitions'

For outpatients, 'urgent' has traditionally meant that the patient needs to be seen within two weeks. 'Soon' patients should be seen within six weeks, and 'routine' patients have no maximum time requirement. For elective surgery, the same terms are used, but there are no agreed corresponding time periods.

These definitions mean very little where waits for patients classified as 'urgent' can be as long as nine months. Reviews of both inpatient and outpatient waiting lists also show that within a waiting list, patients classified as 'routine' frequently wait much shorter time periods than those classified as 'soon' or 'urgent'. There is little evidence that clinical prioritisation affects the amount of time a patient waits.

Prioritisation

Many projects have been run throughout the world to develop more effective methods of prioritisation. Some of these prioritisation techniques, such as those developed in the late 1990's in New Zealand, do manage to prioritise patients in ways that correspond more to clinical need, and some of these methods have been adopted by some Trusts in Britain. Carmarthenshire NHS Trust has also developed a prioritisation system used in other Trusts in the UK with some success.

There is a fundamental flaw in all prioritisation methodology however. As soon as prioritisation is used to ensure that one patient receives treatment ahead of another based on any criterion other than time waiting, some patients will wait longer. 'Jumping the queue', no matter that it is for the best of reasons, means that those at the back of the queue will have to wait longer. The higher the degree of prioritisation used, the longer those at the back of the queue will wait.

Indeed the problem can be worse than just delaying those patients with a low priority. Where there is not excess capacity over the demand, patients with a low clinical priority may *never* be seen — these patients are those at the back of the queue always being 'pushed aside' by those with greater need (see figure 8).

> **GOOD PRACTICE POINT**
> **Prioritisation**
>
> *Clinical prioritisation increases waiting times for lower clinical priority patients. Where clinical prioritisation is necessary, the fewest number of categories should be used. The National Leadership and Innovation Agency for Healthcare recommends using only two categories of prioritization (Urgent and Routine). Points-based systems, or systems with many degrees of urgency, are not recommended.*

Overall, the best way to ensure that all patients wait the shortest *average* time is to have no clinical prioritisation at all, and to see each patient strictly in turn according to when they were added to the waiting list. However, unless there is a very short waiting time, there is always going to be clinical risk if some patients wait too long. In these situations, a level of prioritisation should be used.

FIGURE 8
The danger of excessive clinical prioritisation

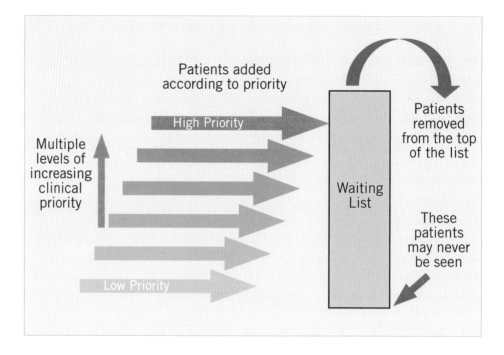

What sort of prioritisation?

The best form of prioritisation, if it must be used, is one with the fewest categories. Prioritisation systems based on complex points systems will add little value, and will take time to administer. The simple, original, 'Urgent, Soon, Routine' is in fact a good degree of prioritisation to use in most situations where there are long waiting times. The NLIAH recommends that only two levels of prioritisation (Urgent and Routine) are used. However, where waiting times are over six months, and there is evidence that a soon category is being used effectively, the 'soon' category can be used as an interim measure.

The key to good prioritisation is consistency of use (from patient to patient, across staff within a department) and ensuring that patients within each category are seen in strict date order. The problem with current systems is not so much the categorisation system used, but the way in which it is used. Prioritising a patient as 'urgent' (i.e. needs to be seen in two weeks) when there is a waiting list of nine months for urgent patients is meaningless and makes the system pointless.

Finally, the important thing to remember about clinical prioritisation is that it is all about patients waiting. Prioritisation, like triage in emergencies, is a way of ensuring that no harm comes to those who have to wait. The best and most reliable way of achieving that goal is to have no waits. If everyone is seen within two weeks, then no-one will have their care compromised by waiting longer than two weeks — irrespective of the method of prioritisation used. The best method of safely and effectively prioritising patients is to ensure that no-one waits.

Clinically Prioritise and Treat Toolkit (CPaT)

No one can argue that patients who are waiting for the same procedure within the same clinical priority should not experience equal waits, regardless of where or who they are referred to. A number of tools throughout this Guide illustrates how to ensure waiting times and the management of those waiting lists are fair to all patients, but how can organisations identify whether their waiting list management is systematically fair? If there are issues, what information do organisations need to inform discussions between the clinical teams, managers and administrative staff to improve the processes for all patients? The Modernisation Agency developed a Microsoft Access® based toolkit to answer these questions.

The Clinically Prioritise and Treat (CPaT) toolkit identifies how waiting lists are being managed by looking at priority category waiting times; procedure waiting times; and the use of statistical process control charts to identify variation in the system. CPaT has been quoted as a "blinding flash of the extremely obvious"[1] as its underpinning concepts are that if routine patients are seen broadly in chronological order, maximum waiting times will reduce, and that the number of patients seen as a priority directly affects the maximum waits for routines.

The toolkit does illustrate variation in waiting times but it does not explain them; its purpose is to stimulate discussions with the whole team as to current waiting list management processes and how to improve them. It does demonstrate potential reductions in waiting times and is designed for different learning styles with a variation in the style of reports that are produced. It produces a system which is fairer to patients, through a locally agreed approach by clinicians, managers and administrative staff. It provides a transparent, systematic and measurable regular monitoring device, measuring improvement in the system and helping to quantify where there are other constraints to reducing waiting times.

The Modernisation Agency have published two guides to assist with the implementation and continual use of the CPaT toolkit: The CPaT Step Guide[2] and the CPaT Toolkit Guide[3]. The former of these is aimed at the CPaT facilitator illustrating what the tools look like and what they show; the benefits and lessons learned from pilot sites; and outlines the steps for local implementation. The Toolkit Guide is aimed at the information professionals to assist with the population of the toolkit. These guides and versions of the toolkit are available to download from the NLIAH website[4]. The toolkit was initially designed to look at inpatient and daycase surgical care, however some of the reports have been locally adapted within Wales to look at outpatient

1 Performance Team, Cumbria and Lancashire Strategic Health Authority as quoted on p8 of the *Modernisation Agency Step Guide: Clinically Prioritise and Treat (CPaT): towards a fully booked NHS.*

2 *Clinically Prioritise and Treat: The CPaT Step Guide.* Modernisation Agency, 2003

3 *Clinically Prioritise and Treat: the CPaT Toolkit Guide.* Modernisation Agency, 2003

4 Some of the following sections within this chapter have been taken directly from the toolkit guides with agreement from the Modernisation Agency CPaT team.

FIGURE 9
CPaT graph
showing long waits
for urgent patients

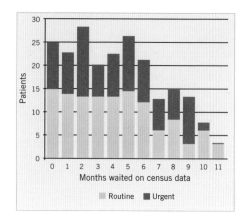

waiting times, and therefore it should be possible to be used through elective care where there are waiting times present.

What CPaT is not:

■ CPaT does not challenge the categorisation of individual patients by clinicians. It presents the information for further discussion within the team.

■ CPaT does not displace clinically urgent patients in order to treat routine patients. When clinical priority is assessed and recorded accurately, seeing routine patients in waiting time order does not interfere with clinical priority patients.

■ CPaT is not a one-off exercise. Like validation, the biggest benefit will occur the first time the waiting list order is improved. Nevertheless, CPaT tools are designed for regular use, to monitor progress and refine waiting list management, and thereby achieve continual improvement.

■ CPaT should not be seen in isolation as providing the answers to waiting list issues, and the reports presented should not be analysed without input from the clinical team and administrative staff. CPaT is starting point for discussions around current waiting list management practices and potential improvement suggestions from staff working within those systems.

FIGURE 10
CPaT graph showing
long 'tail' to routine
waiting list

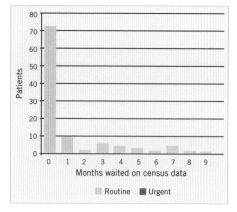

What the CPaT tools look like and what they show:

There are three main charts types of chart that are generated by the CPaT tool:

■ The histogram

■ The rainbow chart

■ The statistical process control (SPC) chart

The different charts will appeal to different people with different learning styles.

The histogram shows patients waiting by months waited and routine patients with an admission date by months waited on admission. These graphs illustrate how long have patients been waiting; are priority patients waiting longer than expected; are routine patients experiencing similar length waits; are routine patients scheduled to be seen in waiting time order; how long routine patients have waited when they are admitted and if routine patients are being seen unduly quickly.

Figures 9 and 10 show a large number of priority patients have long waiting times in the first example, and a large drop in the number of routine patients waiting between zero and one month in the second instance, suggesting that the majority of routine patients are being selected at one month wait, whilst there are routine patients waiting up to nine months. In both cases (and indeed throughout the use of CPaT) further investigation with the clinical and administrative staff is needed.

The Figures 11 and 12 look at how long routine patients will have been waiting when they are admitted: Figure 11 illustrates routine patients being selected for admission within broadly chronological order, as the majority of patients are waiting between nine and ten months for admission. However the figure 12 shows variation in the system for admitting routine patients, showing a wait of between zero and 12 months on admission.

FIGURE 11
A waiting list
managed well

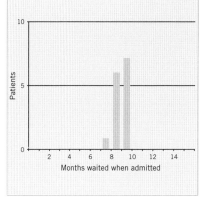

The rainbow charts (figure 13) illustrate whether patients experience similar waits for the same procedure. Currently the toolkit is set to compare the top most common procedures, but this can be reset to reflect local service provisions.

Rainbow charts reflect the clinical indications for the procedure and there is not a single ideal graph. For priority treatments the patients will have been seen quickly, so the red band will dominate the chart, whereas one or two adjacent colours reflecting the maximum length of wait should dominate routine procedures. Where there is a large amount of variation within the system for length of waits there will be few dominant waiting time bands.

FIGURE 12
A poorly managed
waiting list

In the example shown of patients having primary knee replacements, patients treated by consultant one (top band) are not waiting a consistent time but few are waiting over nine months. Many patients are being treated around the two months.

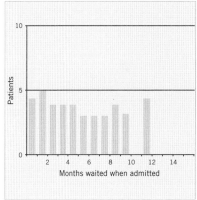

The statistical process control (SPC) charts illustrate the length of wait for individual patients in order of admission (figure 14). This therefore will show the variation in the length of wait for patients; the mean length of wait for all patients and the upper and lower control limits. For further information on SPC analysis see chapter 6.7 within this Guide.

In this example 75 day cases were admitted for varicose vein surgery under one surgeon. The mean length of wait is under $7\frac{1}{2}$ months however many patients waiting under five months have been treated ahead of patients waiting over ten months. The current system of management for this waiting list is producing a waiting time of between one and 18 months.

The SPC reports have been designed to analyse high volume procedures with a relatively predictable rate of clinical deterioration. The procedure groups can be locally set and numbers of patients analysed can be locally limited.

FIGURE 13
Knee replacement
Rainbow chart

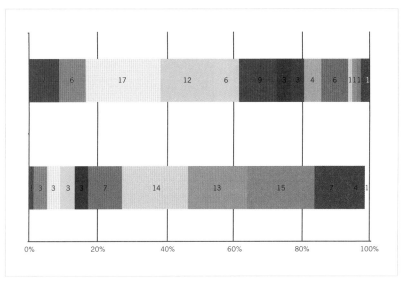

CPaT in Wales:

CPaT has been used in Wales as part of the national *Implementing the Guide to Good Practice Programme*. The main aims of the programme are to ensure all elective patients are treated in chronological order within their clinical priority; to spread patient focussed booking throughout elective care and to redesign in targeted specialties using the tools in this Guide.

FIGURE 14
Varicose vein surgery SPC chart

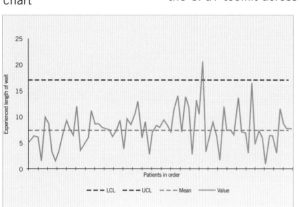

Phase one of the programme was to support all project teams in the roll-out of the CPaT toolkit across all specialties within the organisation for daycases and inpatients. A proposed step plan was presented to the project teams as follows: run and validate reports; meet with Clinical Director and Service Manager to discuss report; meet with individual Consultants to discuss reports; draft action plan and circulate to Consultants and Service Manager for comments; project team to support implementation of action plan and review following implementation within the next specialty. The national programme funded a dedicated project manager and data analyst within each organisation to ensure the prompt roll-out of CPaT and the tools.

Ten months into the programme all organisations were using CPaT to promote discussions with their clinical teams around prioritisation categories, pooling, and validation of their waiting list management practices with the following results:

CPaT in Bro Morgannwg identified inequality in waiting times for some daycase General Surgery procedures. Discussions held with the clinical team supported by CPaT data has generated agreement to pool some General Surgery daycases resulting in waiting times reduced by five months.

The use of CPaT (in particular the SPC charts) in Carmarthenshire resulted in the reduction of prioritisation categories in General Surgery to urgent and routine (with maximum waiting times of 12 months)

CPaT in Ceredigion resulted in agreement to centralise all waiting list management to ensure equity of access and management practices.

Conwy & Denbighshire used CPaT reports to reach agreement to reduce Orthopaedic prioritisation categories to urgent and routine (with maximum waiting times of 12 months) whilst also enabling forecasting of waiting list reductions in Ophthalmology of two months.

North West Wales adapted CPaT reports for on-line real time access by directorates. This information allows teams to drill down to patient level.

CPaT should be used in conjunction with the other waiting list management tools within this Guide to ensure good practice is being upheld and waiting times are representative of a service utilising current available capacity efficiently.

As has already been shown, one of the main causes of long waiting times within the NHS has been the tendency for patients to be treated out of turn. Use of the CPaT tool-kit is one way of facilitating communication between clinicians and managers around ensuring that patients are treated in turn. In this chapter we look at how 'primary targeting lists' can prevent patients being seen out of turn, and how they can reduce long waiting times.

What are primary targeting lists?
Primary targeting lists are simply a way of sorting waiting lists, and a set of procedures for ensuring that patients are removed from the sorted list in order. The system of booking outpatients described in chapter 3 incorporates primary targeting lists, however 'PTLs' should be used wherever a waiting list exists.

Figure 15 shows the consequences of not using primary targeting lists. It shows data from some 500 routine priority patients seen in an outpatient clinic, and illustrates the variation in how long each patient waited.

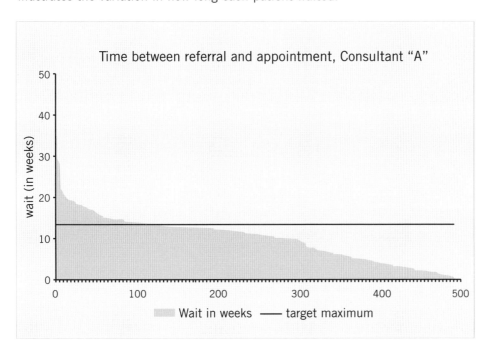

FIGURE 15
Distribution of waiting times

Primary targeting lists are sorted by clinical priority first, and within each clinical priority by waiting time. (Figure 16) Waiting time for sorting the primary targeting list is measured from the *patient perspective*, not the Trust perspective. Sorting within the clinical priority of the PTL is done by subtracting the Clinical Referral Date (CRD) from the current date and ignoring periods of suspension. This calculation ensures that patients are seen in the

Wherever patients are being selected from a waiting list, the waiting list must be prioritised and sorted. Waiting lists should be sorted first by clinical priority, and then by the date the patient was added to the list. Patients should be removed from the top of the list: Longest waiting 'urgent' patients first, shortest waiting 'routine' patients last.

order that they are referred rather than being returned to the end of the list because they have changed their appointment and had their Waiting List Date (WLD) reset. The WLD and CRD have specific definitions detailed on page 19.

This way of ordering of the PTL has some consequences that must be guarded against:

- Where a patient is offered an appointment and is unable to agree to a suitable date, their WLD will be reset. Because only the WLD is reset, and the list is sorted on the CRD, the patient will remain at the top of the PTL. If call in letters are generated automatically, the patient will be called again when the next cycle of letters is generated. Where this is likely to be an issue, it may be necessary to either flag these records in some way or to exclude them from the PTL for a specified period of time. One option would be to suspend such patients for a period of four weeks, and if this can be automated it is probably the best solution as suspended patients will not receive call in letters.

- Where there is picking of patients to avoid breaches of waiting time targets, patients with a long wait measured by WLD will be chosen. This practice upsets the processes described here, however it may be necessary to do this in Trusts with long waiting lists. In this case, sorting the list by WLD may provide a more practical solution. However, the real danger here is that with long waiting times, patients who have their WLD reset will vanish to the bottom of the list and face another, excessive wait.

FIGURE 16
Distribution of waiting times

If sorting by the WLD is undertaken, systems must be in place to avoid this happening.

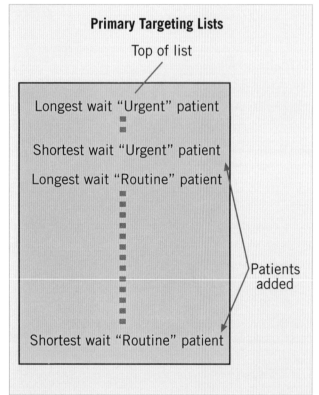

Primary targeting lists are very simple to explain to staff, and easy to administer. They are notoriously under-used despite this. There is a need to put in place monitoring to ensure that primary targeting lists are being consistently used in the administration of all waiting lists. The Welsh Assembly Government has decided that Primary Targeting List Scores (PTLS) must be used as a performance measure of 'treatment in turn' across all elective procedures in Wales. This is covered in chapter 2.7.

PTLs in outpatients and diagnostics
The use of PTLs in outpatient waiting lists is reasonably widespread, and PTLs form the basis of outpatient patient focused booking (covered in Chapter 3). New referrals are sorted by clinical priority, usually 'Urgent' and 'Routine', and then by clinical referral date within each priority. Patients are removed from the top of the list — all 'urgents' before any 'routines'.

This may cause problems where there is a large backlog of 'urgent' referrals. In this case, using the PTL will mean that for a significant period, all clinic slots will be taken up by 'urgent' patients.

Clinically this is an acceptable situation, as the backlog of 'urgent' patients will contain many who have been waiting unacceptably long periods, and it is necessary to sort out the backlog in these categories. In terms of meeting waiting times targets, this process will unfortunately mean that as no patients are being taken from the end of the routine patients, maximum waiting times will increase during this initial period.

To avoid this happening, some Trusts are using a modification of the PTL so that a small number of slots are allocated solely to routine patients, who are taken from the top of the routine part of the list. This goes against the intent of the PTL, but will minimise the increase in waiting times in the short term, and may be a necessary compromise while the backlog is cleared.

Inpatient PTLs

Inpatient and Daycase lists must be managed as primary targeting lists in the same way as outpatient and diagnostic lists. The removal from the list should remain strictly according to list order. Temptations to pick specific conditions to balance theatre time requirements is a constant problem in inpatient lists.

There are two ways of managing this. Where possible, patients should be picked strictly in order from the primary targeting list for pre-operative assessment clinics, and then allocated to surgical lists from those pre-operative clinics (this is described in more detail in chapter 3). Where this is not yet in place, patients should be picked from a band at the top of the PTL, and the make-up of those within the band of patients monitored closely to ensure that no patient remains within the band for any length of time. This allows surgeons a 'restricted flexibility' around who they choose for surgery. Monitoring of Primary Targeting List Scores will help this process.

GWENT HEALTHCARE NHS TRUST

Monitoring outpatients

Measures were required to provide information about the performance of waiting lists. It was important to gather enough information on a regular basis to assess how modernisation strategies and capacity were affecting lists.

A number of measures were developed and were provided centrally to directorates. They are distributed monthly to Directorates.

The measures include:

1. *Booked activity against template (to monitor under and over activity)*
2. *New to follow-up ratio and breakdown of priority (changes)*
3. *DNA rates by priority (monitor reductions and increase)*
4. *Cancellation rates*
5. *Average waiting times per Consultant and site (shows variation)*
6. *Waiting times by waiting band — by month (shows variation and reduction of 'tail')*
7. *Primary target rates (selection of patients from the back)*
8. *Primary target list score (selection of patients from the back)*
9. *Total list scores (change in waiting times measured in days not patients)*
10. *Referrals*
11. *Rate of partial booking*

The measures and results have generated interest and development in three areas.

1. *Pooling across Gwent — Variance in average waiting times and poor primary target rates have generated interest in pooling as a means of improving waiting times.*
2. *Tidying up data — common problems include erroneous prioritising of patients and multiple referrals.*
3. *Increased understanding of template variance — this has encouraged closer monitoring.*

Where there has been a practice of picking from well down the list to fill surgical lists (e.g. day case patients in orthopaedics) the problem is not one of managing the PTL, it is instead a problem of imbalance in the provision of inpatient and day case lists. In this situation, adjusting the balance of daycase work to inpatient work, or moving more work onto the daycase list, is preferable to maintaining unequal waiting times.

Prioritisation of inpatient PTLs

Unlike the outpatient PTLs, there may be a need to prioritise patients more carefully on inpatient lists. The coarse prioritisation into 'urgent' and 'routine' may not be adequate for inpatient lists that are long. There may be patients who are 'routine' but cannot wait as long as the most 'routine' case.

Additional levels of prioritisation such as a 'soon' category are acceptable in this situation, but should be used with care. As has been described in the prioritisation section, the more levels of prioritisation used, the longer the waiting times will be for the most 'routine' cases. Where there is a greater flow onto the waiting list than off it (and consequently the list is getting longer) high degrees of prioritisation will ensure that some patients at the back of the list never receive surgery — and certainly not within the target times set by the Assembly.

Monitoring primary targeting lists

The use of primary targeting lists is erratic, even in Trusts where their use is policy. The development of a good monitoring tool that both ensures the use of PTLs and shows their impact on waiting lists, is essential. In 2003 a team in the Gwent Healthcare NHS Trust developed two measures, the Primary Targeting Rate (PTR) and the Primary Targeting List Score (PTLS). The PTLS is now officially recognized as a performance management tool by the Welsh Assembly Government, and is described in Chapter 2.7.

GWENT HEALTHCARE NHS TRUST

Measuring primary targeting

*Primary targeting lists were used extensively in Gwent to reduce outpatient waiting times, with significant results. One of the reasons the use of PTLs was so successful was the development of key measures by the improvement team in the Trust. Two of these measures were the **Primary Target Rate** and **Primary Target List Score.***

These two measures were used throughout the Trust in monitoring the reduction in maximum waiting times for new outpatient referrals. Both measures are described in detail in 2.7, and the NLIAH would like to acknowledge the work of the Gwent team in developing and promoting these measures.

In 2005, the use of the PTLS was mandated by the Welsh Assembly Government as a measure of efficiency in managing waiting lists, and it is now used across all waiting lists in all Trusts in Wales as a performance measure.

Monitoring PTLs: the PTR and PTLS

One of the problems associated with ensuring good waiting list management practice is that there have been no clear and simple measures that show whether a particular waiting list is being managed appropriately. For this reason, the *Implementing the Guide to Good Practice Programme* adopted Primary Target Rates (PTR) and Primary Targeting List Scores (PTLS) as measures of whether patients are being treated in chronological order. This chapter describes the two measures, how they are calculated, the issues associated with their use, and how they can be used to manage waiting list performance.

The introduction of 'Patient focused booking' (including partial booking) has meant that treating patients in chronological order has become far more prevalent in the making of first outpatient appointments. In 2003 Gwent Healthcare NHS Trust developed the PTR and PTLS as a way of presenting the impact of partial booking on outpatient waiting lists. These two measures provide simple, easily calculated, single figure measures of how well routine patients are being removed from the end of the waiting list. The *Implementing the Guide to Good Practice Programme* is extending the principles proven in outpatients to inpatients, day cases, diagnostics and therapies. The PTLS is being used as a core measure to judge the impact of the programme.

The Primary Target Rate (PTR)

The *Primary Target Rate* is a simple measure that illustrates the ratio of the number of patients treated from the end of the waiting list to the number of patients who could have been removed if all were removed from the end of the list. The calculation of the PTR is quick and simple:

- Add all patients treated during the month to the waiting list at the end of the month.

- Sort the list into clinical priority order, and then chronological order within each clinical priority.

- Count the number of routine patients who were treated during the month. This figure is the denominator of the ratio (A).

- Count (A) places down the sorted routine list from the longest waiting patient and mark this point.

- Count how many routine patients who are above this point have been removed from the waiting list this month. This is the numerator of the ratio (B).

- The PTR is B/A expressed as a percentage.

The PTR is quick to calculate, but is a coarse measure. With small number of removals and picking of patients around the margin of the list it is possible to have fairly effective waiting list management with a low PTR. For this reason, we recommend the PTLS as a performance measure.

A theoretical case is shown in figure 17. There are 100 patients on the waiting list. 25 patients have received treatment during February 2005. We therefore draw a line 25 patients down from the top, and count the number of treated cases within that top 25 (there are 14).

FIGURE 17A
Calculating the PTR
Step 1
Count down from the top
of the list

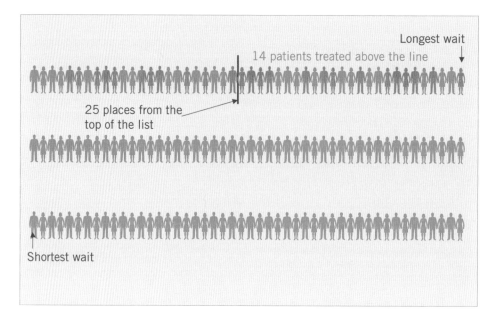

The PTR is therefore 14/25 x 100, or 56%.

FIGURE 17B
Calculating the PTR
Step 2
Doing the calculation

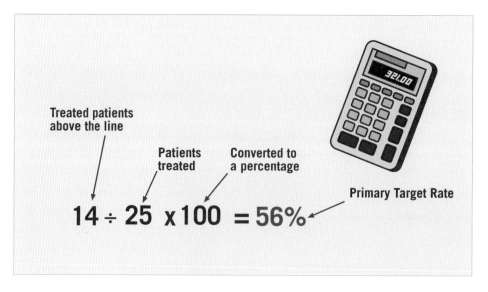

The PTR will show a low score if there are many patients treated below the line, even if those patients have been waiting a similar time period as those above the line. Additionally, the PTR does not discriminate on the position of those below the line — picking a patient from the bottom of the list (waiting a few days) has the same impact on the score as picking a patient from just below the line. This is shown in figure 18, where there are two lists which give the same PTR, although the top list exhibits quite good treating in turn, while the second list does not. For this reason the NLIAH recommends the use of the PTLS rather than the PTR.

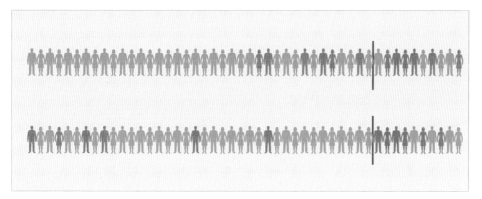

FIGURE 18
The PTR does not
distinguish where the
patients were
removed from

The Primary Targeting List Score (PTLS)

The *Primary Targeting List Score* is a more complex ratio that takes into account the time a patient has spent on the waiting list. Instead of the position on the list, the number of days on the list is used for the calculation. It therefore distinguishes between picking patients close to the line and picking patients from the bottom of the list. It is also less sensitive to selection just above and below the line, giving a greater degree of clinical freedom in the making up of operating lists.

Two figures are required to calculate the score, which is the ratio of the number of days waiting removed from the list in the month (the numerator) to the maximum number of days that could have been removed (the denominator). The **numerator group** refers to all patients who were removed, the **denominator group** refers to all patients on the waiting list (whether used in the calculation or not).

First, as with the PTR, add all patients treated during the month to the waiting list at the end of the month.

Before undertaking the calculation, all urgent cases must be removed from the list. Although the best approach is to not have a 'soon' category, at this time it is also acceptable to remove patients from the list who are prioritised 'soon'. This should not preclude working to eliminate the soon category.

Remove all 'special category patients'. These may include patients seen in nurse led clinics and paediatric cases for some specialities. Be careful about allowing these removals — there must be a very sound reason for the decision (see below for these two examples).

Remember that no patient can appear in the numerator group and not appear in the denominator group.

Patients who are booked into a clinic or session and DNA should be removed from both the numerator group and denominator group. Patients who have, through the application of patient focused booking, agreed a date past the end of the calendar month, should also be removed from both the numerator and denominator group. Their booking will be counted in the following month PTLS calculation.

- Once all the necessary removals from the list are complete, identify all the patients treated during the month. For each patient, calculate the number of days they waited (Operation date minus the WLD or CRD, depending on which measure you are using. WLD if used for performance management, CRD for internal use). Add the total number of days waiting for this group. This is the **numerator**.

- For each patient on the waiting list at the end of the month who does not have a booked appointment, calculate the number of days the patient was on the list at the middle of the month (the 15th day of the month minus the date treated). This gives the effect of averaging the potential for removal as if patients were removed evenly across the month.

- Sort the list by the WLD or CRD (WLD if used for performance management, CRD for internal use).

- Count down the number of places from the longest waiting patient that is equal to the number of patients in the numerator group. Add the total number of days waiting for this sub group. This is the **denominator**.

The PTLS is the numerator number of days divided by the denominator number of days, expressed as a percentage.

Figure 19A-D show the process using the same set of data as before. The total number of days on the list for those treated in February is 8470. The total number of days that *could have been removed* (the top 25 patients) is 9729. Therefore the PTLS is 8470/9729 x 100, or 87%.

As can be seen from this example, it is possible to get a score above 80% even though there were only just over 50% of the patients treated within the top 25. This is because no patients were taken from the lower part of the list; although the list was targeted imperfectly, in general patients were removed from the back of the list, not randomly throughout. This is one reason for choosing the PTLS rather than the PTR; it rewards good behaviour rather than just perfect behaviour.

Issues in calculating the PTR and PTLS

There are some issues that need to be taken into account when calculating the PTR and PTLS.

Should you use the CRD or the WLD?

Chapter 2.2, *Understanding the Definitions*, describes two 'start dates' for waiting list events (page 19). The first, the CRD is used to order the PTL for purposes of ensuring that patients do not wait unnecessary lengths of time. The CRD is fixed at time of referral and never changes. The second, the WLD is not fixed, as it may be reset when a patient fails to attend an appointment, or changes their appointment date repeatedly.

As already explained, the reasons for having two dates is to separate performance issues from patient choice. If a patient chooses to cancel or not attend, the WLD may be reset, so that calculations of waiting time do not unduly penalise the Trust. However, it would be unfair to drop such a patient back to the bottom of the waiting list when waiting times are so long (in some situations adding a further 18 months to their wait) so as far as possible we should use a list sorted on the CRD as the pick list for making appointments.

Where the PTLS is being used as a performance reporting tool, it is only fair to the Trust that PTLS calculations are based on the WLD (the performance measure date), not the CRD. This will ensure that Trusts are not penalised for targeting patients who are potential breaches of waiting list targets. However, Trusts should in this situation calculate both scores to fully understand what is going on in the service.

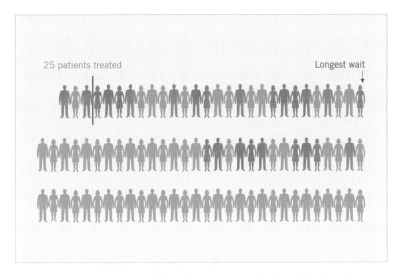

FIGURE 19A
Calculating the PTLS
Step 1
Count down from the top
of the list!

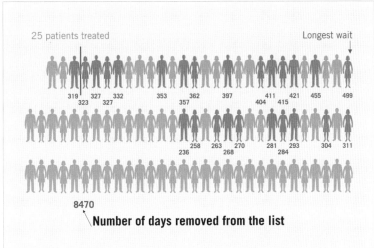

FIGURE 19B
Calculating the PTLS
Step 2
Add the total wait of the
treated patients

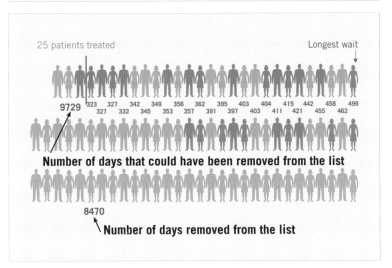

FIGURE 19C
Calculating the PTLS
Step 3
Add the total wait for the
top 25 patients

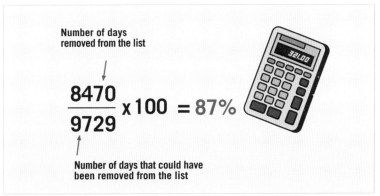

FIGURE 19D
Calculating the PTLS
Step 4
Doing the calculation

What about Nurse led clinics?

Nurse led clinics will pick patients from the consultant waiting list based not on time, but on the competency of the nurse. This means that nurse led clinics can substantially reduce the PTLS if these patients are included.

If the patients had been allocated to the nurse waiting list at time of referral, and were treated in order, there would be less of a problem. However it is still likely that the maximum waits are much shorter, and this would reduce the speciality PTLS. This is a similar effect to that reduced by pooling, however pooling cannot be applied across consultant / nurse boundaries, so does not apply.

The correct way to treat the nurse clinics is to report the PTLS for that clinic, but *exclude* the nurse clinics and patients from the speciality score. Remove these patients from the list before it is sorted and do not include the number seen in nurse clinics in the total removed from the list.

What about paediatric patients?

In some specialities, children are selectively removed from the waiting list out of order for clinical reasons. Where this is justified for clinical reasons, the cases removed should be treated in the same way as nurse led clinics ie the patients should be removed from the waiting list before any calculations are undertaken.

Using the PTLS as a performance management tool.

There will always be some variation around the scores due to clinic needs and patient choice. For this reason it is unwise to use a high degree of precision in comparing scores. In performance reports that the NLIAH prepares for the Welsh Assembly Government, we round all scores to the nearest 10% before reporting and work to an agreed 'target PTLS' of 80%. The flexibility this gives will allow for issues of patient choice and clinical freedom without adversely affecting performance to the target.

It is important to remember that the PTLS not only measures whether patients are treated above or below the nominal line, but also from how far below. Low scores usually represent picking from well down the list, rather than just flexibility around the margin.

For Trusts with small numbers of patients removed each month, variability is likely to be more of an issue. For this reason it it may be better to calculate the PTLS on a 3 month rolling average, rather than each individual month. This will buffer the impact of relatively small discrepancies in picking having large impact on scores, due to the small numbers of cases involved.

Reporting on the PTLS should initially be done at speciality level. However, it is possible to have a situation where every consultant (or site) is reporting a high PTLS but the score for the speciality is low. This is due to a lack of pooling, and the effect can be seen in figure 20.

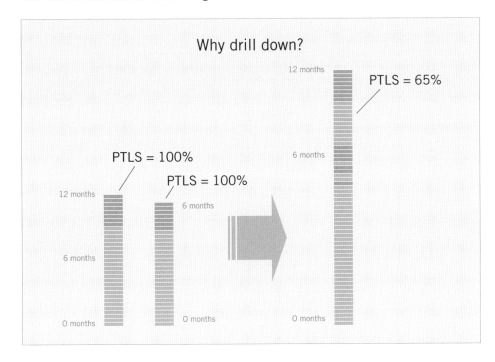

FIGURE 20
Example
Calculating the PTLS
for the combined list

In the figure there are two waiting lists, each with patients removed from the top. List A has a maximum waiting time of 370 days, and the PTLS is 100%. List B has a maximum waiting time of 121 days, and a PTLS of 100%. However, if the total list for the speciality is calculated, the 10 patients removed from list B come from further down the combined list:

In the combined list, it can be seen that there is no longer 100% removal from the top of the list; in fact the PTLS has now dropped to 65%.

If the two lists were pooled (across consultants, across two sites) then the lists would be better managed and the combined score would rise. Once again, it is not to be expected that pooling will be 100%, so setting a target score of 80% allows for imperfections in pooling. Pooling is covered in more detail in chapter 3.2, and in many places in Wales pooling is now in place for many specialities.

Patient focused booking

3

Booking is integral to improvement in the NHS in Wales. This chapter will look at a number of different aspects of booking, dealing with the full range of inpatient and outpatient events. The total approach to booking is referred to as *Patient focused booking*, and this phrase should be used whenever possible. Above all, avoid use of the phrase 'partial booking' when communicating with the public.

Why patient focused booking?

The NLIAH recommends that all appointments between patients and Trusts be made by agreement. In some cases this means that appointments are made while the patient is present (for example some follow-up outpatient appointments) while in other cases it means that appointments are made by telephone. In some cases it will mean that an appointment with another health provider is made at a previous appointment — for example, a secondary care outpatient appointment may be made while the patient is at their GP.

Patient focused booking: A combination of full booking, direct booking and partial booking

Full booking

In England, policy requires that Trusts move towards a policy of full booking with choice. The key principle for full booking is that the patient leaves an appointment knowing the exact date and time of their next attendance at the Trust. In fact, this is common for follow-up appointments in most Trusts now.

Full booking requires a date to be negotiated with the patient no matter how far into the future an appointment will be. If the waiting list for a particular surgical priority is nine months, then under a full booking system, a date for surgery must be agreed for nine months into the future.

With a six week policy for leave it is not possible to give the patient a reasonable assurance that the Trust will not have to cancel an appointment made several months into the future.

Partial booking

Partial booking has been included as part of patient focused booking by the NLIAH because it enhances patient choice, ensures clinic and theatre efficiency by reducing non-attendances and cancellations, and improves communication between the Trust and the public.

GOOD PRACTICE POINT
Patient Focussed Booking

All appointments where the patient attends the Trust should be booked. The key requirements of patient focussed booking are that the patient is directly involved in negotiating the appointment date and time, and that no appointment is made more than six weeks into the future.

Partial booking differs from full booking in one key respect: no appointment is ever made more than six weeks into the future. With a six week agreed leave policy, the need to cancel appointments or surgical dates is significantly reduced. It is possible to give a strong assurance that an agreed appointment will be honored by the Trust.

CONWY & DENBIGHSHIRE NHS TRUST
Nurse practitioner ophthalmic service

The needs of the ophthalmic patient have dramatically changed over the past decade. Changes and advances in computer and surgical technology, lasers, drug therapies, digital imaging and so forth have changed ophthalmic practice unrecognisably and the delivery of ophthalmic services has changed to address these demands. Technological advances have increased public expectation of patient and health service provision. Waiting is no longer an acceptable option.

The development of the Nurse Practitioner role has evolved to include management of nurse-led glaucoma clinics and postoperative cataract clinics. Safe practice is assured through competency-based training, clinical supervision, mentorship and an induction programme. An advanced educational module for nurse practitioners is also available in North Wales and co-ordinated locally at H. M. Stanley hospital in St. Asaph. All practitioners adhere to agreed clinical pathways of recognised practice, with documentation and patient outcomes regularly monitored through audit. In addition to nurse-led clinics the practitioner team is responsible for diabetic retinopathy screening in the local community and the assessment and treatment of specified ophthalmic casualties.

Practitioners have played a vital role in assisting the Directorate to meet annual targets for referral waiting times, casualty services and nurse-led services. Feedback is gathered formally from service users in the form of user surveys, which provide feedback and favorable support for practitioner input.

Direct booking

Direct booking has been a major focus of booking in England. Electronic booking is a key to the English implementation of direct booking.

Direct booking involves GPs having access to Trust appointment systems so that they are able to book appointments within the Trust from their surgery while the patient is present. In Wales, direct booking is recommended as part of patient focused booking, as long as the appointment being booked is no more than six weeks into the future. The NLIAH does not recommend direct booking more than six weeks into the future.

Electronic booking, as an enabler of direct booking for urgent appointments, is part of the Informing Healthcare strategy[1].

1 *Informing Healthcare* Welsh Assembly Government 2002

Generic referrals and pooling

Traditionally in the NHS, referrals have been made from a GP to a named consultant. Patients seeing a specific consultant have been placed on that consultant's waiting list. Patients seen in one location are followed up in the same location. Patients seen on one site will have their diagnostic procedures performed on that site. Patients will be seen in specialist or subspecialist clinics. All of these factors increase waiting times, and all can be addressed through generic referrals and pooling.

What are waiting lists?
Staff tend to think of waiting lists as an indication of a shortage of resources, but resource shortage is not the only reason waiting lists develop. Waiting lists are simply queues, and a lot can be learnt about managing waiting lists from how other organisations manage queues.

Understanding queues
Queuing theory is a well developed science in mathematics, and fortunately one does not need to understand it in depth in order to make progress on managing waiting lists. The one thing it is important to know is that a single queue in front of multiple 'windows' will have shorter overall waiting times than a series of short queues in front of each window. This is the 'Post Office' queue, seen in most commercial premises apart from supermarkets.

The basic unit of the queue is the primary targeting list described in the previous section. Rather than each consultant having a single outpatient waiting list, there should be a single list for the speciality. Rather than multiple inpatient waiting lists, each surgeon should pick from the top of a single list. Eventually, outpatient and inpatient lists should be managed as a single process on a single list. This is the same as having a single queue in a bank, and the customer going to the next available window.

Problems with pooling
Unfortunately, waiting lists are not bank queues. There are multiple priorities within waiting lists, and there are multiple subspecialities within a speciality. Multiple priorities within a list are easily managed through the use of PTLs, as illustrated in Chapter 2. Management of subspecialisation is more of a problem, but it is one that must be resolved. There are three possible solutions.

Maintenance of a 'pooled' list
The simplest solution to the problem of pooling in subspecialities is to maintain a generic pooled list in addition to each consultant's own subspeciality list. All patients who need to be seen within a subspeciality are added to the individual

---

GOOD PRACTICE POINT

Generic Referrals and Pooling

Referrals into Trusts should be pooled within specialities. Referrals to a specific consultant by a GP should only be accepted when there are specific clinical requirements, or stated patient preference.

consultant list, while those able to be seen by any consultant are added to the pooled list. The main problem with this approach is ensuring that the pooled list is treated at the same level of priority as the individual lists. In most situations where this approach has been used, consultants exhibit a tendency to remove patients from their own subspeciality list ahead of those from the pooled list. In some cases it has been found that patients are added to a pooled list and no-one removes them.

'Hidden' pooled lists

A solution to this problem can be to 'hide' which patients are on generic lists and which are on the subspeciality lists. This solution is the best option where it can be implemented electronically, or where waiting lists are maintained centrally. It is harder to co-ordinate where each surgeon or their secretary maintains the list.

FIGURE 21A
Step 1: Three different lists

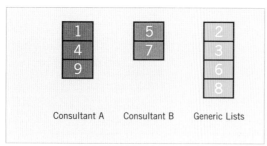

In this method, separate lists are maintained on the IT system, one for each subspeciality and one for the generic patients. Patients are added to the bottom of each list. (Figure 21A.)

When the lists are displayed, the subspeciality lists are merged with the generic list in referral date order. Patients from the generic list (the yellow cases in figure 21) are shown on each list. The patients have not been added to both lists — they still exist on a third actual list, so they are not duplicated although they appear to be. They are simply shown in the new 'virtual' lists as demonstrated in figure 21B.

FIGURE 21B
Step 2: Combine the lists

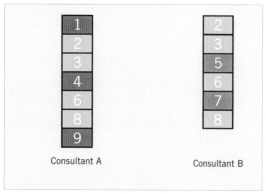

When the lists are displayed, it is important not to distinguish on screen between the generic patients and the subspeciality patients. Each consultant will see a single waiting list of their own patients merged with the generic patients, with no visible distinction between the generic and the subspeciality patients. (Figure 21C.)

The reason that this method works best when implemented electronically or through a centralised waiting list management team is that otherwise there is the possibility for a patient to be picked from the list by more than one consultant. In an electronic system using virtual lists, record locking protocols will prevent multiple picking, while in a centralised environment management procedures can be put in place to have the same effect.

FIGURE 21C
Step 3: The consultant view

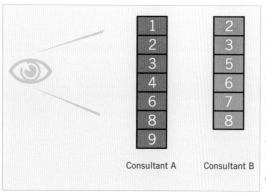

The Matrix approach

What if it is not possible to implement a generic list either electronically or centrally? What about situations in large Trusts where there may be multiple consultants in each subspeciality, making the implementation of the 'Hidden Pooled List' more complex? A number of Trusts use an approach of adding each new referral to the shortest waiting list, using a matrix to determine which waiting lists are available.

The first step in this approach is to sit down with the clinical staff in the speciality and list all the conditions on the waiting list, and all the staff available to see or treat those patients. A matrix is then constructed. (Figure 22A.)

Then, with the involvement of the clinical staff, each cell of the matrix is filled in so that every condition has at least one consultant marked. Where there is not a consultant, it must be determined who is available to see those patients, or what the Trust policy is for managing those patients. There must be no blank rows on the matrix. (Figure 22B.)

Each row of the matrix can now be considered as a 'clinical care group', that is a group of patients who can be managed by a specific group of clinicians. Some consultants may appear in several clinical care groups with different colleagues. (Figure 22C.)

Each consultant will have their own entirely unique waiting list. The patient is added to the shortest waiting list within the clinical care group. In the example in figure 22D, a patient with condition 3 will be added to Consultant AA's list, because that is the shortest waiting list out of AA and DD, the only two waiting lists in the matrix for condition 3. (Figure 22D.)

What do we mean by shortest?

There are many definitions of 'shortest' when describing waiting lists. Each has potential problems.

Fewest patients on the waiting list

This definition does not take into account the rate at which patients are removed — a consultant who operates on a lot of complex cases will take patients off the waiting list at a slower rate. A consultant who has many outpatient clinics will remove outpatient referrals at a faster rate than one who has few clinics.

Shortest Wait

The consultant with the shortest maximum waiting time may seem a sensible definition of shortest, but it is defining shortest future wait on the basis of shortest historical wait, and will not take account of changes in circumstances. This will be most clearly seen in cases where most consultants have a wait of 12 months, and a new consultant starts work. By definition, that consultant will have the shortest wait (under 12 months) for the first year, and potentially all patients referred in that year will be added to that list — leading to an inflated list for one consultant which may take some time to clear.

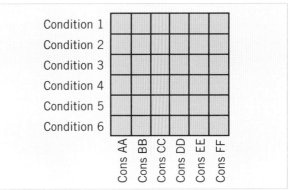

FIGURE 22A
Step 1: Create the matrix

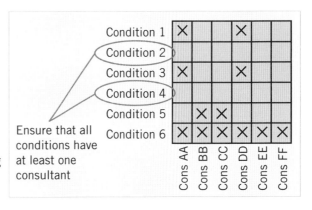

FIGURE 22B
Step 2: Fill in the matrix

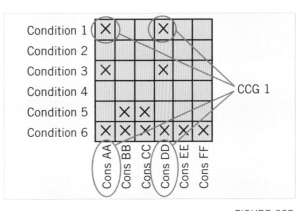

FIGURE 22C
Step 3: Identify the Clinical Care Group

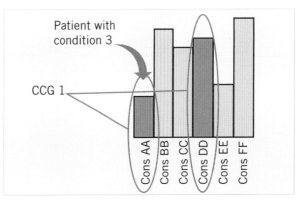

FIGURE 22D
Step 4: Select the shortest list

Clearance Time

A better definition, which is prospective rather than retrospective, is clearance time. This is calculated on the basis of the number of patients on the waiting list divided by the rate at which patients are being removed. The clearance time in weeks is the number of patients on the list, divided by the number expected to be removed each week. In effect, this is the time that it would take to clear the list if no new patients were to be added, or the time that a patient added today could be expected to wait.

Clearance time will only be accurate as long as circumstances do not change, but will be adjusted automatically if circumstances do change. It does take some account of casemix on the list, as casemix will affect removal rates. Counting on the basis of casemix would be even more accurate however.

CARDIFF AND VALE NHS TRUST
Pooled waiting lists in Cardiology

This initiative was taken in response to the need to address differential and unacceptably long waiting times for cardiology outpatients referred to the Trust's 6 consultant cardiologists.

A detailed consultant-led review was undertaken to determine how this situation could be addressed. This resulted in a plan to pool all referrals for agreed conditions. Waiting lists for both Trust sites were merged, and booking templates agreed for all clinics so that the same number of patients is planned for each.
A protocol was agreed with consultants for assigning referrals to subspeciality clinics only on an exception basis, with all others being considered as suitable for the pool. In each consultant clinic, a certain number of slots are set aside for subspeciality patients, with the remainder of the slots being used for patients from the pool. The consultant who sees the patient at their first appointment undertakes any subsequent follow-up. The system was designed to be compatible with partial booking.

The new system achieved a reduction in numbers of patients waiting over 18 months between January and March 2003 from 188 to just 13. By April 2005 maximum waiting time of 13 months had been achieved.

Counting casemix rather than patients

Chapter 5.3 points out the danger of counting work as patients or Finished Consultant Episodes (FCEs). When calculating clearance time, it would be useful to allocate an expected theatre time for the condition to each patient on the list, so that the clearance time can be calculated in theatre minutes. This will be far more accurate than any measure that works on patient numbers.

Who owns the pooled list?

There is one final question: who has clinical responsibility for a pooled or generic list? It is a requirement of the Welsh Assembly Government that every patient waiting for either inpatient treatment or on an outpatient list is allocated to a specific consultant in terms of clinical responsibility. Where a matrix approach is used to allocate patients to lists, generic or pooled lists do not exist so this is not an issue. Where 'hidden' pooled lists are used, or even the simple pooled lists mentioned first, there needs to be a named consultant for the pooled list.

In most cases in Wales, the Clinical Director of the service has taken on responsibility for the pooled list and is recorded as the named consultant.
The important thing to keep in mind is that the named consultant for a pooled list has responsibility for the patient while they are waiting. Once the patient has been booked for surgery with a consultant, they become that consultant's responsibility.

Pooling will have its biggest impact when there are significant differences between the length of waiting lists (either by consultant or site). Where lists are relatively even, the effect of pooling on waiting times will be less. However, the use of pooling and generic referrals is good practice, and should be encouraged even when the impact on waiting lists would be minimal.

Why generic referrals?

Generic referrals are referrals sent to the Trust, rather than a named consultant. In most cases, the referral will be to a 'Dear Doctor'. Generic referrals are good practice. They recognise that the Trust delivers a service, not solely the consultant, and they allow the Trust and primary care to determine how the service should best be provided (either pooled consultant lists, or alternative practitioners). Generic referrals will promote equity of access as waiting times will be based on the date referred rather than the consultant referred to.

Cost savings will be found when the use of generic referrals means that patients can be seen by staff other than a consultant. For example generic dermatology referrals could be seen by a GPSI rather than the consultant. This will reduce the cost per case, allowing greater volume through the system.

GWENT HEALTHCARE NHS TRUST
Caerphilly Back Pain Pathway

The Back Pain Pathway started on 1st October 2002 following funding from Caerphilly Local Health Group. It offers GPs within Caerphilly Borough an acute access service for patients with low back pain. The team is headed by an Extended Scope Practitioner (ESP) and senior physiotherapists, supported by technical and administrative staff. Patients access the pathway via GP referrals made against set criteria and are then paper triaged by the ESP, (usually within 48 hours of referral).

Patients with complex conditions are assessed and treated by the ESP or referred on appropriately to main stream physiotherapy, a back education and lifestyle programme, Pain clinic, or Radiology for further investigations as required. There is direct access to an Orthopaedic Consultant should any patient present with serious pathology or require a surgical opinion.

This pathway offers a comprehensive integrated service to GPs allowing patients with low back pain to be seen promptly by the most appropriate practitioner at a location most convenient to them.

Between 1st October 2002 and 31st August 2003 a total of 869 patients were referred to the Pathway. Of these, only 1 was referred to the Orthopaedic Consultant and 1 was referred to Radiology.

The pathway has improved quality of patient care, with 88% of patients reporting satisfaction with the waiting time for their first appointment, 75% showing an improvement in their condition with physiotherapy and 96% of patients being satisfied with their treatment location.

The Problem

Surgical outpatient waiting lists had inequality between three consultants — waiting times varying from two weeks to 13 months. The consultants, who sub-specialize (ie breast, vascular and colo-rectal), would not accept a generic waiting list for outpatients. Despite this, GPs often have very little idea about 'who does what' in the hospital.

The Solution

1. *Ask the consultant with the longest waiting times if he would consider transferring any patients to the other consultant's lists. Ask the other consultants if they will see the transferred patients.*

2. *Trawl through all of the longest waiting list with the consultant to see who could be transferred.*

3. *Send letters to both the patients and their GPs asking if they want to be transferred and thus be seen sooner, with an option to stay with the original consultant if they so wish.*

4. *Draw up a matrix of conditions and get each consultant to acknowledge which he will see as an outpatient, and subsequently as an inpatient or day case.*

5. *Inform the GPs of each consultant's waiting times for first outpatient appointments, day case surgery and inpatient lists, together with the matrix of conditions. Inform the GPs on a quarterly basis of the waiting times as above.*

The Results

97 patients were deemed suitable by the consultant to be transferred. The other consultants agreed to see them. Out of the 97 only 13 patients were not transferred either at their or their GPs request.

The 84 patients were all seen within six weeks.

The consultants supported the matrix and informing the GPs of their individual waiting times. The matrix was only given to the GPs at the beginning of August and so there are firm numbers to report. However, on looking at the outpatient waiting lists at the beginning of September it appears that the two consultants with shorter waiting times have had more referrals in August than the previous months. It will be easier to establish whether it has had an impact after 3 months. The Trust is hoping to introduce this method of keeping GPs informed for all specialities in the future.

The booking process

This chapter deals in detail with the booking process: how and why partial booking works, how to apply it to returning outpatients as well as new referrals, how patient focused booking can be used to ensure that cancer patients are seen within ten days, and how booking works with inpatients and day cases.

Patient focused booking basics

Partial booking is an unfortunate phrase that has become common currency within Trusts, but which should be avoided when communicating with patients. The NLIAH recommends the phrase **Patient Focused Booking**, which incorporates the entire booking process. This document defines partial booking as part of the overall booking process.

Partial booking is not, in itself, a form of booking. It is a way of managing the waiting list to ensure that when booking takes place, it is done with the direct involvement of the patient. Partial booking is a set of processes and procedures to manage the waiting list (such as the integration of primary targeting lists into the PAS letter generation process); a set of principles around patient booking (such that no appointment is made without the direct involvement of the patient either by phone or in person); and a set of practices, such as the use of appointment centres to provide a single and central point of contact for patients within the Trust.

The relationship between partial and full booking is shown in figure 23 on page 62, but it can be reduced to a very simple rule: if the appointment is going to occur within the next six weeks, then full booking should be used. If it is going to be further than six weeks into the future, then partial booking should be used.

Why patient focused booking?

There are three main reasons for abandoning the old system of appointments. Patients are not seen in order; patients do not have a choice of date and time when receiving their appointments; and a lot of time is spent cancelling appointments. Patient focused booking addresses all of these issues.

Patients are seen in order

Patient focused booking uses clinical priority and time on the list to calculate when a patient will be seen. This is a considerable improvement on the essentially random allocation of appointments that has happened in the past. The patients who need to be seen within six weeks are booked directly into appointment times through direct booking. Patients who are not able to be seen in six weeks are placed onto a list which is sorted first by clinical priority and then by waiting time. The sorting of waiting lists is covered in more detail in chapter 2.6, Primary targeting lists.

FIGURE 23
An overview of the
booking process

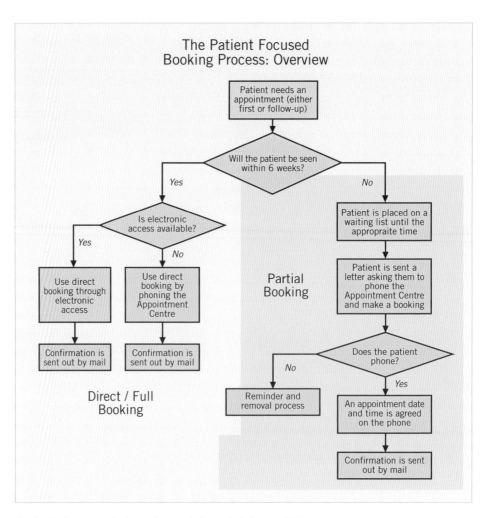

The Patient Focused
Booking Process: Overview

Patient needs an appointment (either first or follow-up)

Will the patient be seen within 6 weeks?

Yes — Is electronic access available?

No — Patient is placed on a waiting list until the appropraite time

Yes — Use direct booking through electronic access

No — Use direct booking by phoning the Appointment Centre

Partial Booking

Patient is sent a letter asking them to phone the Appointment Centre and make a booking

Confirmation is sent out by mail

Confirmation is sent out by mail

Direct / Full Booking

Does the patient phone?

No — Reminder and removal process

Yes — An appointment date and time is agreed on the phone

Confirmation is sent out by mail

Patients have a choice of appointment date and time

Patient non-attendances and patient cancellations consume a vast amount of resource, as well as severely affecting the flow of patients through clinic (as shown in chapter 1). By agreeing a date and a time with the patient, either face to face in the case of direct booking or over the phone in the case of partial booking, the incidence of cancellations and DNAs because the appointment is booked for a date or time that the patient cannot attend is considerably reduced.

When the patient is arranging their appointment at a time that suits them approximately four weeks into the future, they are far less likely to forget their appointment. This will further reduce DNAs. DNA rates have dropped from 14% to 3% in some clinics where patient focused booking has been introduced, and most clinics achieve the target rate of less than 5%.

Hospital cancellations reduce

Because the Trust has a leave policy requiring six weeks notification of any leave that will affect an outpatient clinic, and because the clinics are only filled approximately four weeks before they happen, clinics which are cancelled for routine reasons (annual or study leave) will be cancelled at a point when there are no patients booked into them. No patients need to be cancelled, and no re-work is necessary. The few cancellations at short notice (e.g. due to sickness) can be rescheduled into an empty clinic in five weeks time.
Less re-work means more staff time available for other duties.

Partial Booking: New referrals over six weeks

The partial booking process is illustrated in figure 24. The process acknowledges the referral when it is received, and sends letters to patients four weeks before they need to attend, asking them to phone and make an appointment.

FIGURE 24
Partial booking flow diagram

The acknowledgement letter

As a patient is registered and prioritised, a letter is generated telling them the approximate wait, and telling them to expect another letter closer to the time. An explanatory leaflet on the process is enclosed with the first letter. A sample letter can be found on page 78.

If the patient is to be seen within 6 weeks, they are asked to phone straight away and make an appointment. These are patients that should be seen through the direct booking process, but have been referred in as a lower priority or because the GP does not want to use the direct access route.

Generating the 'Pick List'

Every week, staff look at clinics for four weeks ahead. For each clinic they calculate how many patients will be needed to fill the clinic, and select those patients from the top of a 'pick list'. The pick list is sorted first by priority order, then referral date order.

The 'Phone' letter

The 'picked' patients are each sent a letter, which asks them to phone the Appointment Centre as soon as possible to arrange a suitable date and time for their appointment. When they phone, an appointment is made on the PAS and a confirmation letter is printed and sent.

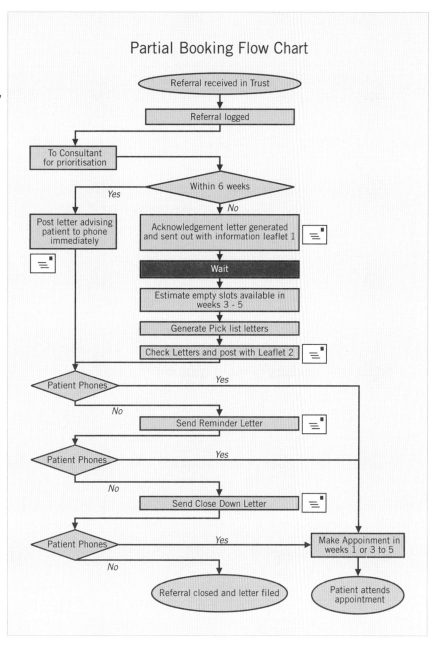

Partial Booking Flow Chart

The system is 'self balancing'. If too few patients phone in any week, extra letters can be generated the following week. Similarly, if more patients phone, bookings can be made into week five, and correspondingly fewer patients 'picked' the following week.

A reminder letter is generated automatically for those patients who do not respond to the 'phone' letter. If they do not respond to this reminder within two weeks, the referral is automatically closed and a letter is sent to the GP as well as the patient.

Partial booking: Follow-up bookings over six weeks
There are considerable advantages to be gained by applying the methodology to follow-up outpatients as well as new referrals. Cancellation and DNA rates are usually higher for follow-up patients than for new referrals. Clinics are frequently overbooked with follow-up appointments because these patients are perceived as having a higher clinical priority than new referrals. In specialities where 'mixed' clinics (containing both new and returning patients) are common, all the benefits of partial booking will not be seen until all patients are booked using patient focused booking.

There are different issues involved in partial booking for follow-up patients. New routine referrals are seen on a 'first come, first served' basis within clinical priority. With non-urgent follow-up patients there is usually a clinically significant time in which they should be seen. We cannot see the two week postoperative follow-up in ten weeks, or the 12 month review patient in six weeks. For this reason, partial booking for follow-up patients is implemented in a slightly different form. This involves a calculation of priority when generating the pick list, rather than a sort of the pick list on the basis of assigned clinical priority and then waiting time.

Some Trusts in England have tried prioritisation of patients based on required appointment date. This means that at the start of June, the list will show patients due for appointments in July. This works where there is adequate capacity for the service — but if there are more requests for appointments than there are available appointment slots, then the patients will be called later and later after the requested time. If requested appointment date is the sole prioritisation criterion, limited appointment slots may not be made available to those who need them most. While some patients may be able to wait two months from the requested date, others may not. A patient who should be seen in twelve months may safely be able to wait fourteen months. A patient due to be seen in two months may not be able to wait four. If this system is used, the monitoring process described at the bottom of page 143 is necessary.

While no prioritisation system will resolve a mismatch between capacity and demand, where there is a mismatch it is important to prioritise the patients to make best use of the limited resources. This suggested solution takes account of the 'flexibility' that may be present in longer time period appointments.

1 Define the 'Appointment Delay'
Two dates need to be provided: the Request Date RD (when the appointment was requested) and the Target Date TD (when the appointment should occur).

2 Calculate the acceptable range
Two further dates are now determined: calculate the delay TD — RD, then set the Start Date SD (TD — 20% of the delay) and the End Date ED (TD + 20% of the delay). These two dates define the acceptable range for the appointment. Note that because a percentage is used, longer interval appointments e.g. 12 months will have a larger acceptable range than shorter interval appointments e.g. three months.

3 Assign a priority
At the time the pick list is generated, a priority must be assigned. This is recalculated each time the pick list is generated, because the priority is determined by the relationship between the clinic date CD (the date for which the pick list is being generated — usually four weeks into the future) and the dates above.

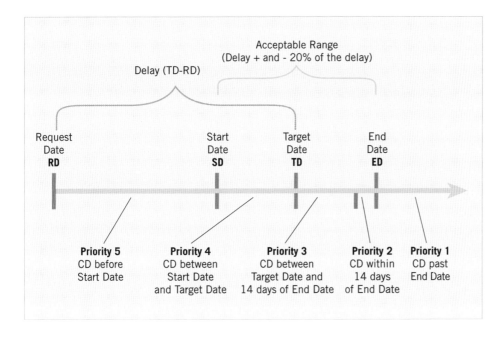

FIGURE 25
Prioritisation of
follow-ups

Priority One
The Clinic Date (CD) is after the End Date (ED). This means that the appointment is already overdue, beyond the acceptable range of possible appointments.

Priority Two
The Clinic Date (CD) is within 14 days of the End Date (ED). This means that unless the appointment is made immediately, the clinic will fall outside the acceptable range of dates.

Priority Three
The Clinic Date (CD) is after the Target Date (TD), but not within 14 days of the End Date (ED). This is an acceptable position for the appointment to fall.

Priority Four
The Clinic Date (CD) is before the Target Date (TD), but it is after the Start Date (SD). This is an acceptable position for the appointment to fall.

Priority Five
The Clinic Date (CD) is before the Start Date (SD). There is no point in making this appointment, as the patient will be seen before they need to be.

4 Pick the patients
Pick the patients to send for in order of highest priority (One is high) first, then within the priority order, by Target Date.

Using the pick list as a monitoring tool
A useful consequence of the prioritisation system is that it gives continuing feedback on the capacity available for return appointments. If priority One or Two patients are appearing consistently in the pick list, the demand for appointments exceeds the capacity and more must be made available.
If there are any priority Five patients picked, there is too much capacity, and some resources should be diverted to seeing more new patients.

Direct booking: Appointments within six weeks
Because there is a six week cut-off, appointments cannot be made into clinics further than six weeks into the future, and so partial booking is used.
Within six weeks from now it is possible to guarantee a clinic and direct booking can be used.

Direct booking for new referrals
There are two circumstances that apply with new referrals. One, the preferred situation, is called GP direct access booking and it is covered shortly.
The second is where the referral is received through the normal 'non-urgent' mail referral, but the GP has marked the letter urgent or the consultant has upgraded the referral to urgent. As already described these patients are sent a 'phone us now' letter through the Appointment Centre, and are in other respects handled as if they were a partial booking referral. The exception to this case is those patients who fall within the 'ten day' rule — primarily cancer referrals. These are dealt with separately on the following pages.

Direct booking for follow-up patients
This is almost the trivial case of direct booking, as it is no change from the traditional practice. Where a follow-up appointment is required within six weeks, it is made in person at the reception desk before the patient leaves the clinic. The only difference from traditional practice is that the appointment will be easier to make — because the clinic will not be clogged up with long term follow-ups already booked in some months earlier.

GP direct access
Allowing GPs direct access to booking systems will provide a greater degree of confidence to the GP and the patient that they are being appropriately cared for by the Trust. While GP direct access may be based on technology, there is also the option of implementing GP access through existing phone technology by use of the appointment centre.

The flow chart in figure 26 illustrates how both full and partial booking would work under either system.

The NHS in Wales is not currently trying to achieve a system where all outpatient appointments are booked by the GP. Because there is a system in place that means no patient is booked over 6 weeks into the future (partial booking), GP access to clinics with waits over 6 weeks will result in registering the patient for partial booking rather than allocating a specific appointment time.

One of the advantages to direct access booking is that it allows short notice appointments (under six weeks) to be allocated at the time that the patient is in the GP practice, reducing both time and work at the Trust. Another advantage is found if an automatic process is put in place to provide feedback to GPs on the referrals they make — this is covered in Chapter 9.5 under 'GP Feedback'.

Booking 'urgent cancer' patients
The Welsh Assembly Government has a requirement that certain categories of patients (primarily some patients with suspected cancer) are seen and treatment commenced within target times. Booking systems must be set up to ensure that these patients will be seen within the required time.

FIGURE 26
GP referral process

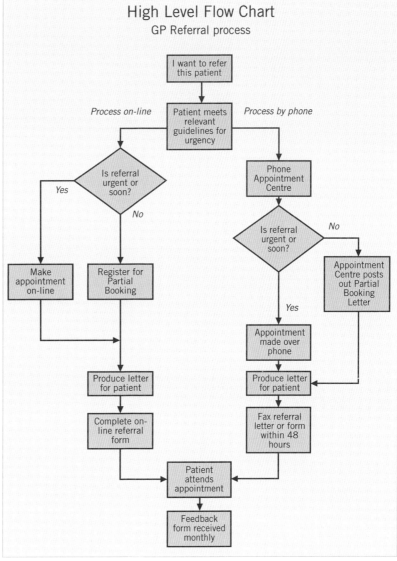

One of the problems in meeting the requirements of the guarantee involves ensuring that there are enough appointment slots for these patients every week. Normal booking processes attempt this by setting aside an average number of slots for urgent and cancer referrals. This does not work.

FIGURE 27
Average and adjusted maximum cancer referrals

Some weeks there are not enough slots...
Because the clinics are planned for the average, there will be some weeks when there are not enough slots. If this is an isolated week, or if the clinic did not have to adhere to a ten working day standard, there would not be a problem — patients would be

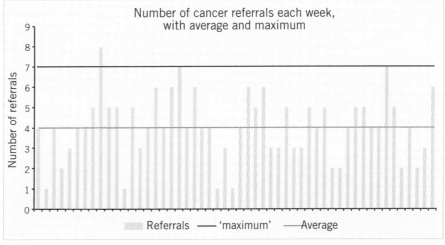

booked further ahead, and it would 'all average out over time'. With the ten day standard, a couple of weeks of higher than average referrals will breach the standard.

Some weeks there are more slots than patients...

As with the 'too many patients' problem, there will be some weeks, or a run of weeks, with too few patients to fill the available slots. Because the number of slots is based on the average number of referrals, using these vacant slots at the last minute eats into the supply of slots, yet if not used, they are wasted — the next referral cannot be booked into a slot last week just to 'average' the clinics out!

What is the solution?

The problem is one of allowing adequate slots for a 'run' of above average referrals, yet not wasting slots by providing more slots than there are referrals. The challenge is to provide this without overbooking or underbooking the clinic — the right number of patients arriving at every clinic.

One approach to this problem uses the Appointment Centre and patient focused booking. The number of slots each week is set to almost the maximum referrals received in any week (actually to the 80th percentile). This sets aside more slots than there will be patients most weeks. The NLIAH recommends using data from a full year for this calculation. (Figure 27)

FIGURE 28
Booking 'urgent cancer' patients

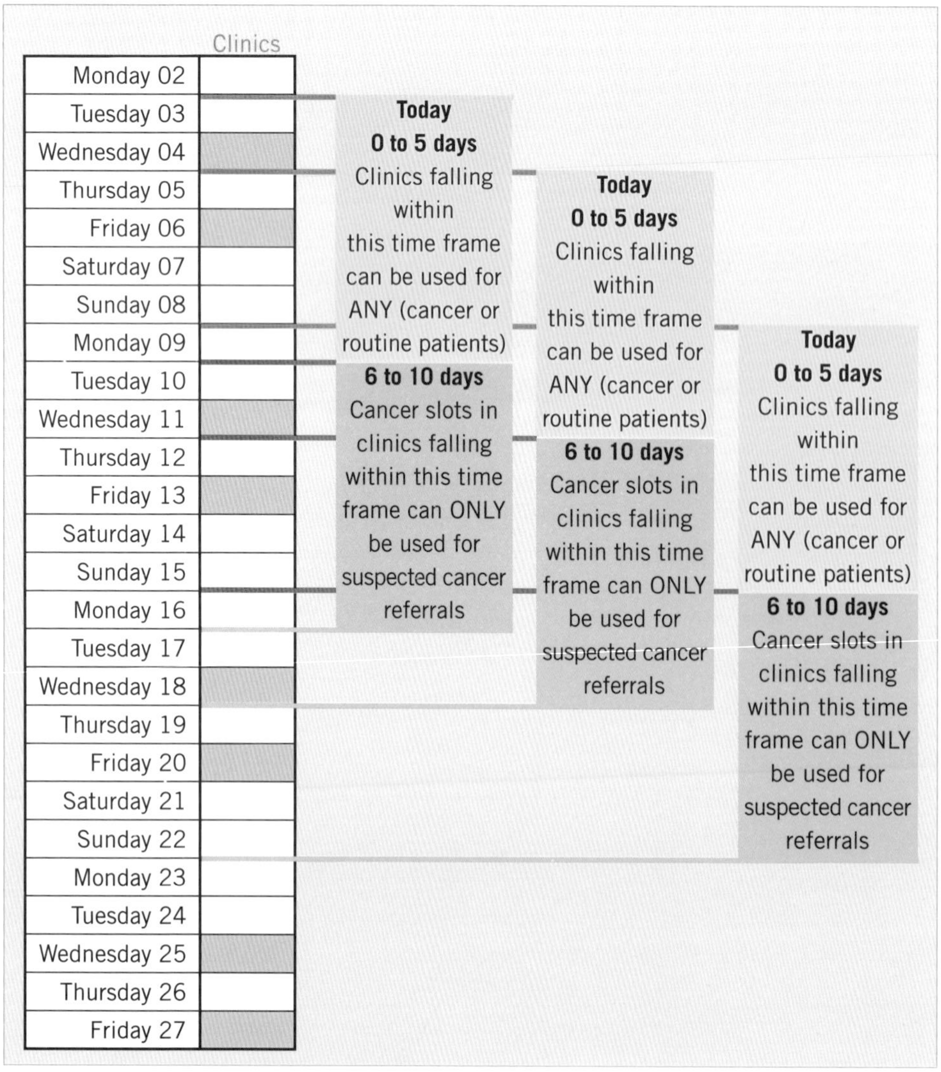

Any vacant slots in the current week are filled with routine patients, or other GP referrals, if there are no ten working day referrals. There is no danger of breaching the ten working day wait rule, as there will almost certainly be enough slots next week for however many patients are referred, even if all this week's slots are filled.

Because there are always patients phoning for appointments, slots not used during the preceding week can be filled. The process is described diagrammatically in figure 28. The template shown includes two clinics per week (Wednesday and Friday, shaded) and a calendar is shown for four weeks.

The first column shows the situation on the first Tuesday (3rd). The cancer slots in the two clinics that fall between six working days and ten working days (the clinics on the 11th and 13th) are strictly reserved for cancer patients only. The slots in the clinics between today and five working days (the clinics on the 4th and 6th) may be used for any cancer referrals, but they may also be used for any other patients who phone for appointments — even if they are routine appointments.

Two days later (on Thursday 5th) the situation has changed. The time periods are now shown in the middle column. The zero to five working day period (reversed) now includes the clinic on Wednesday 11th, and any cancer slots in this clinic are now available to be filled by any patient who phones in. The loss of those slots to cancer referrals is compensated for by the fact that the clinic on the 18th is now available for cancer bookings.

The following week, the situation has changed again (third column). Once again, the clinics within zero to five days (those on the 11th and 13th) are now available for any referral, while those in the 6 to 10 day frame (18th and 20th) are reserved for cancer patients only.

The moving template will continue to slide on through the month — always reserving at the very least one full week of clinics within the ten working day deadline, yet back-filling any slots not used by day 5 with any referral.

Where this system is in use it is possible to ensure that all patients are first seen within ten working days, without wasting capacity or overbooking clinics.

Patient focused booking, inpatients and day cases
The system of booking outpatients described above cannot simply be extended to inpatients or day cases. Appointment Centre staff are unlikely to have the expertise or access to information needed to make up theatre lists, which will require matching groups of patients with varying length procedures to make best use of skill mix, equipment and time. Yet the benefits of patient focused booking will be even more significant in booking theatre lists where the costs are so much higher than outpatient clinics.

Booking as a two stage process
The best approach to booking for inpatient and day case surgery is to treat it as a two stage process. First book the preoperative assessment, and then book the actual surgical date at the preoperative assessment.

The Preoperative assessment appointment
Where the patient is to receive surgery within six weeks of being placed on the list, the preoperative assessment should be completed at the time of the outpatient appointment. In many Trusts this is done within the day surgery unit or on the appropriate surgical ward, and the patient is directed there from the outpatient clinic.

Where the wait is longer than six weeks, the patient is listed in the normal way and advised of the likely wait. The preoperative assessment is then treated as if it was an outpatient appointment. An appointment is booked for a preoperative assessment in a clinic run on the ward or in the Day Surgery Unit. This is booked using the partial booking process through the Appointment Centre.

Because the assessment is likely to be relatively generic, there are none of the problems of booking the appointment directly for theatre.

Preoperative assessment clinics can be booked for a range of theatre lists. It is not necessary for all patients on a list to be booked into the same assessment clinic. 'Phone in' letters for the assessment clinics can be generated on the basis of an 'average' flow through to the actual theatre list, as the actual matching of patients to lists can be done at the preoperative assessment when the patient attends in person.

Arranging surgery at preoperative assessment

When the preoperative assessment is completed and the patient is clearly fit for surgery, the list can be booked. There will be a range of theatre lists over the next six weeks available to the person doing the booking, and if necessary the booking could be made slightly further into the future. Because the staff doing the assessment are also doing the booking, the issues of casemix on the list do not apply — the specialist knowledge required is held by the preoperative clinic staff.

In some cases it may not be necessary for the patient to attend for a preoperative assessment. In these cases, an assessment may be carried out over the phone.

FIGURE 29
Booking Inpatients and
Day Cases Overview

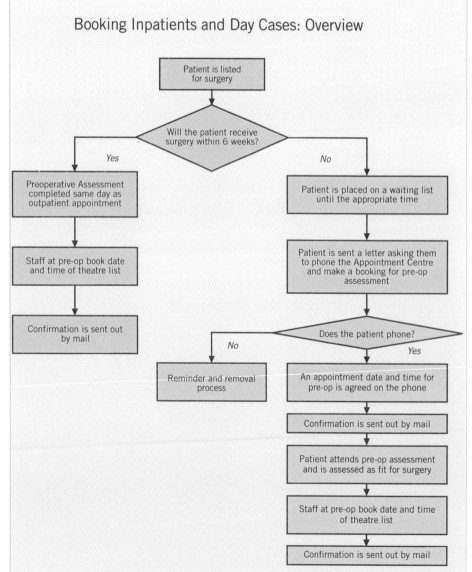

Telephone preoperative assessment

Telephone assessment is best done by writing to the patient and inviting them to contact the appropriate department at a date and time convenient to themselves within a given range, eg. Monday to Friday between 2pm and 6pm.

On contacting the department the patient is asked a series of questions, and is either deemed fit to proceed to negotiate a date for admission and surgery, or it is felt that the patient will need to attend for outpatient preassessment and therefore the date for this will be negotiated with the patient whilst on the phone.

At the time of the telephone call, the date and time for surgery are agreed as if the patient were present at the preoperative assessment clinic.

A flowchart of the whole process can be found in figure 29. The booking of preoperative assessment clinics and the impact on theatre performance is covered in more detail on page 81.

Partial Booking in Diagnostics and Therapies

Diagnostics and Therapies fall between the simplicity of booking outpatients and the complexities of booking theatre lists. In most cases, the lists will be able to be booked through the Appointment Centre as long as particular attention is paid to the setup process and training Appointment Centre staff to deal with these more specialised clinics.

One specific problem that may be seen is that many services have no access to the PAS, or use a computer system that is independent of the PAS. This means that many of the issues seen in the early stage of setting up outpatient booking will need to be revisited. Either partial booking capabilities will need to be put into the existing diagnostic computer systems, or a link will need to be made to the PAS. Where systems are manual, they will need to be set up as PAS clinics, which will involve some network and equipment issues.

Designed for Life[1], the strategy document for the NHS in Wales, sets the NHS waiting time targets based on total waits from referral to treatment rather than the traditional approach of separate lists and targets for surgical waits and outpatient waits. As the NHS changes to these targets, integrating booking systems with those in the main clinical specialities is essential. Too often in the past problems in diagnostics and therapies have been overlooked, but that is now changing.

Implementing patient focused booking

Patient focused booking will lead to significant reductions in DNA rates and cancellation rates. As many consultants have taken DNA rates into account when calculating clinic sizes, an important step in introducing patient focused booking must be to review the clinic profiles.

Step 1: Meet with the medical staff

There is less potential for confusion amongst staff if patient focused booking is introduced speciality by speciality, rather than consultant by consultant. This means that clerical staff in the medical records area do not have to decide whether a generic referral has to go to the new or the old process. Staff in clinics, who may need to answer questions about referrals, will be less confused. Overall the change will be smoother.

It is important to approach each consultant individually. Avoid working solely through third parties, such as a Clinical Director. A group meeting with the consultants in a speciality may be an alternative if individual meetings are not possible, but ensure that a follow-up meeting is arranged with any staff not present. There are a few outcomes that must flow from the meeting.

1 *Designed for Life, Creating world class Health and Social Care for Wales in the 21st century.* Welsh Assembly Government, 2005

Adherence to a six week leave policy

You must get the agreement of the consultant staff that they will adhere to a six week notification of leave policy. This is essential. In changing the system, you are removing some apparent certainty for the patient in return for far greater certainty that their appointment will not be cancelled. Without agreement from consultant staff that they will not cancel clinics at short notice, you are unable to give that certainty to the patients who phone in. This is the only concession that you will require from the consultant staff, and most will see it as a small imposition — in fact, there are likely to be only a small number who do not do this already.

The notification period must apply to the junior staff as well — in fact, to all staff whose absence would lead to the cancellation or reduction in size of a clinic. In general, consultant staff are much better at adhering to this policy than are junior staff. This may reflect the fact that we are poor in communicating with junior staff due to regular rotation, and it will be useful to ensure that this policy is covered in any orientation material sent out to new staff.

One reason for short notice cancellation by junior staff is that leave is applied for in another run or hospital, and the staff arrive in a new department with pre-approved leave for the next week. Good communication and orientation practices should reduce this problem.

Of course, having the agreement of staff to adhere to a six week policy will only work if the processes are in place to ensure that leave notification is promptly acted upon. It is essential to have clear leave approval procedures that ensure clinics are able to be closed off within a few days of the leave being requested, otherwise clinical staff who adhere to the policy will still see clinics cancelled, but for purely administrative reasons. A clear policy backed up by good and prompt procedures will make the process work.

Clinic profiles

Consultant staff must review their clinic profiles. The new profiles must assume there will be no DNAs. Do not accept an assurance that the profiles are OK — review them anyway. This is likely to be the most time consuming stage of the process.

Implementation timetables

Ensure that all staff understand that the new system will not have an effect until all patients currently booked into the system are seen. A common misunderstanding is that the patient focused booking is not working because clinics are over booked six weeks after the meeting — but the clinics were booked up 12 weeks ahead, and are still working under the old system.

After the meeting, send a letter to each consultant thanking them for their time, reconfirming the six week rule, the commitment to review the clinic profiles (with a date for the first draft) and a date by which the clinic should be operating fully.

Before working on profiles, it will be useful to meet with the nursing and clerical staff for the speciality. The purpose to the meeting is to explain the new booking system to them, and to get any information they may have on quirks of the clinics. Once again stress how the new system will resolve current problems, and aim to get them enthusiastic in support of the changes. Dissatisfied staff in the clinic can do a lot to sway the consultant staff against change, and staff who are on board will help with the minor problems that will arise during implementation.

Start from the existing clinic lists — not the booking rules on the system, but the lists of actual attendances in clinic. Often the clinic profiles on the system bear little resemblance to the actual booking rules, which may exist solely in the heads of the consultant and clerk.

Determine how many slots need to be reserved for urgent patients — based on how many patients attend within seven days of referral. How many acute patients are seen? How many soon? Are the clinics made up of new and follow-up patients, or are there separate clinics for new patients? Analysis of the clinics for the past few months should give a good starting point for this information. Determine both the average figure and the maximum in any particular clinic — it is important to determine whether there is much variability in types of referral, or whether the referral rates are predictable.

FIGURE 30
The Appointment Centre
in Conwy and
Denbighshire Trust

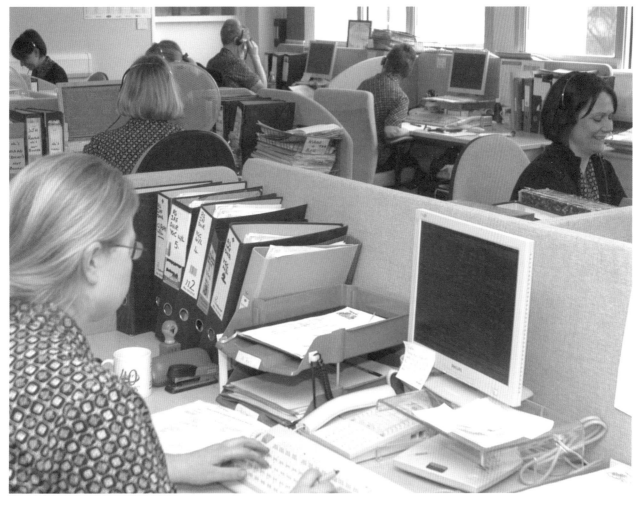

Some patients need help getting to their appointment. This transport is organised by the GP practice once an appointment has been made by the Trust. The cost of transport is met, not by the GP, but by the Trust.

This system causes a number of problems. Often transport is booked too late, and the patient DNAs. Frequently an appointment is cancelled, but since transport is arranged through the GP practice, no one knows to cancel the transport. GP practices spend a lot of time arranging the transport. There is no accountability between the Trust and the GP when one organisation is paying and the other does all the ordering.

With the Trust Appointment Centre making partial booking appointments, there is an opportunity to fix these problems. Patient transport bookings should be made by the Trust Appointment Centre at the time the appointment is made. Use of a clear script to elicit whether transport is required will reduce unnecessary use. The transport booking should be recorded on the PAS, so that if an appointment is cancelled the transport can also be cancelled.

This system reduces transport 'DNAs', and Trust DNAs caused by failure of the transport process. It reduces the cost to the Trust of patient transport. It eliminates the need for the patient to contact their GP to arrange transport, and it reduces workload in GP practices who no longer have to be involved in the process.

One concern about the use of booking is that the system will increase costs. It is true that there are more mail costs, and in some cases extra staff may be needed in appointment centres.

There are ways to reduce the costs however. Many staff are involved in printing, checking and enveloping appointment letters at present, and there are also mail costs involved in the current system. One potential solution being investigated by Trusts in England and Wales involves forming a partnership arrangement with an outside contractor to print and process the letters.

In this system, letters are sent electronically to a print bureau, who sort the electronic file by postcode, print and despatch the letters. The sorting of the files means that Trusts can take advantage of Royal Mail discounts on postage, and less space and capital expenditure is taken up by printers and enveloping machines. Where Welsh language is required, the use of fast duplex printers allow the printing of English and Welsh on opposites sides of the page, again reducing cost.

It is also possible to use the checks in this system to reduce wrongly addressed mail.

Avoid 'carve-out' caused by allocating too many 'slot types'. Reduce the number of types of slots to a basic four: new referrals under two weeks; new referrals over two weeks; follow-ups under six weeks; follow-ups over six weeks. See page 141 for more detail on carve-out.

Once the booking rules are drafted based on this information, confirm them with both the consultant and the clinic staff as being workable. Remember that they must not include any assumed cancellations or DNAs. Also check that the number of new referral slots will allow the Trust to see the number of patients referred. Be careful of allowing clinic numbers to drop significantly unless there are clear reasons why the clinics were previously overbooked. It is important to not create a problem of reduced capacity through this process.

Finally, set up the new profiles on the system to start from the date that you have determined all previously booked patients will have been seen.

Step 4: Start patient focused booking for this speciality

The system 'goes live'.

Step 5: Review the booking rules

Once patient focused booking is implemented, and several clinics have run where all patients have been booked through the new system, go back and meet with the staff again to determine whether any changes need to be made to the booking rules. It is quite possible that there were perceived problems that have led to under booking, or that insufficient slots were removed to allow for the reduction in DNAs.

Step 6: Diary dates for regular review of the booking rules

Things change. Don't assume that getting things right the first time will mean that the booking rules are set in stone. All clinic profiles should be reviewed at the minimum annually. This review should include start and finish times, the number of new and follow-up slots, and the timings of appointments. The review should be conducted as part of the process of balancing annual capacity and demand, so that increases or decreases in demand over the year can also be addressed.

CONWY & DENBIGHSHIRE NHS TRUST
One stop clinics including pre-operative assessment

In response to the ongoing quality development programme in Ophthalmology it is now common practice for patients to attend their new letter clinic appointment, be placed on the surgical waiting list and undergo preoperative assessment all within the same visit.

It is recognised that for most referrals, the reason for referral may be identified. The patient is therefore sent an information booklet regarding the condition they are referred with prior to their appointment. This process provides the patient with sufficient opportunity to be informed before their appointment.

This practice meets with best practice recommendations and is evidence of improved efficient and effective patient preparation preoperatively to reduce cancelled surgical cases at short notice. The objective of preoperative assessment clinics incorporated at listing in the clinical area is to provide efficient delivery of ophthalmic services to the patient in an informative manner. Careful planning and health education processes provided during this process enables the Directorate to plan duty rosters, skill mix and full theatre utilisation.

One-stop clinics for surgical listing take place daily at H M Stanley hospital, and are planned at Colwyn Bay and Holywell peripheral clinics. The success of these clinics is dependent on resources and skilled ophthalmic staff supported by well co-ordinated clinic bookings.

Future aims to improve this service will be to expand technical resources available such as biometry, focimetry and keratomery equipment to increase potential throughput.

The service provides patients with their admission date at this assessment, when anaesthetic support is available for all theatre lists.

It is planned to include all peripheral clinics in this one-stop service to provide true equity of services in the NHS in our catchment area of North Wales.

Setting up an Appointment Centre

The heart of the patient focused booking system is an efficient phone centre. Avoid the use of the term 'call centre' as it sometimes has negative connotations, but there is no doubt that the system depends on a dedicated team of staff who can accept calls and make appointments.

Setting up a centre is no different than it would be in any other industry, and it is useful to benchmark your service with call centres from outside health. The requirements are simple:

FIGURE 31
The Appointment and Booking Centre in Cardiff and Vale NHS Trust

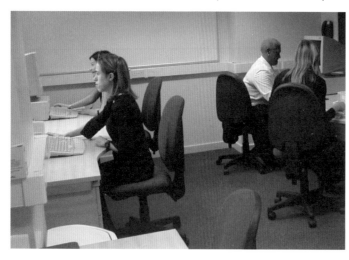

1 Location

The Appointment Centre must be somewhere where mail access for external (referral) mail and internal mail is delivered several times a day. While in theory it is possible to site the centre anywhere, proximity to the trust will make communications simpler.

2 Equipment

Dedicated phone lines are essential. These should have a single number for the public to call, feeding into multiple operator lines. Look into the availability of specialist equipment — eg call distribution software that randomly allocates calls to the operators, headsets to allow hands free operation, and phones which allow staff to complete transactions on their computers before accepting another call.

FIGURE 31
Making and appointment in North West Wales Appointment Centre

3 Staffing

The Appointment Centre should be staffed for extended hours and staff need to be employed on contracts that allow shifts to cover these times. Full training of staff will be necessary.

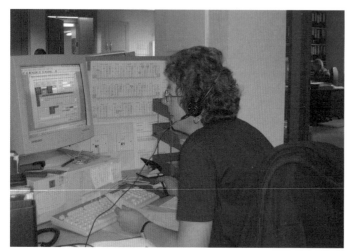

4 Training

The Appointment Centre is as much the public face of the Hospital as the Accident and Emergency Department or the Outpatient Clinic. For the majority of the public accessing the services of the hospital, the Appointment Centre is likely to be their first contact with a hospital staff member. For this reason it is extremely worthwhile to put time and energy into the public relations skills of the Appointment Centre Staff.

Several Trusts in England and Wales use a training programme with an external agency who specialise in telephone skills, covering all aspects of dealing with the public by phone. The programme, spread over four half day sessions, has been tailored to the specific problems and questions likely to arise in a call centre dealing with patients.

New Surgical Super-Clinic at H M Stanley

Mr Andrew Maw leads the first surgical super-clinic at the Trust. The first clinic was held on Friday the 18th February, and utilises the whole of the General Outpatient Department at H M Stanley on a Friday afternoon.

The lead consultant, a specialist registrar, an SHO, two nurse endoscopists, one nurse practitioner, two pre-assessment nurses and two stoma care/colorectal nurse specialists make up the team.

Any patients attending the clinic who require surgery will be pre-assessed for fitness for surgery and given information regarding their surgery with the process of informed consent starting while they are there. The nurse endoscopists will manage their caseload of new patients and provide treatment and follow up for those with benign disease. The stoma care/nurse specialists are present for advice and counselling and they conduct a nurse led stoma and colon cancer follow up clinic.

A rapid access nurse-led flexi scoping service is planned as an extension to this clinic and is set to commence shortly.

New Patient Appointment Centre at Glan Clwyd Hospital

The Trust opened a new Patient Appointment Centre based at Glan Clwyd hospital at the end of 2004.

The new centre introduced Patient Focused Booking at the Trust for acute specialties. This new booking process offers patients greater choice regarding the date for their appointment, so they are involved in deciding a mutually convenient time. The quality of the service to the patient is improved by providing greater certainty that the date they are given will take place, and need not be changed.

Patient Focused Booking fixes all the problems caused by patients who DNA (did not attend), and the re-booking caused by cancelled clinics and patient cancellations. Because the patient is arranging their appointment at a time that suites them, and for a period within four to six weeks, they are far more likely to attend. DNA rates have dropped in Wales from 14% to 3% in many clinics, and evidence from patient satisfaction surveys nationally indicate that patients like the new way of arranging their appointment.

Mrs Debbie Hogg, the new Patient Appointment Centre manager, is well known for her experience in training users on the Trust PAS system, and is an expert in clinic management and templates. Early indications of success show drops in waiting times for clinics, and a happy response from our patients when they are asked which date is convenient for them.

By April 2005 the following DNA rates were achieved:

ENT	4%
Elderly Care	1%
General Surgery	5%
Oral Surgery	5%
Oncology	2%
Ophthalmology	1%
Paediatrics	4%
Rheumatology	3%
Dermatology	6%

Acknowledgement letter (sent after prioritisation)

Dear

I have received a letter requesting an appointment for you to see a consultant in **Specialty.**

A consultant has seen the letter and asked us to make you a 'non-urgent' appointment.

The current waiting time for this kind of appointment is ... months. **(If the waiting time will be longer than 6 months include the following:** We are very sorry that you will have to wait this long for your appointment. I can assure you that we are doing everything we can to reduce our waiting times). The Trust has passed your referral to the most appropriate consultant team. If you request to see a specific consultant, your waiting time may increase, and maximum waiting time guarantees may not apply.

Because we will need to write to you about your appointment, please remember to phone us if your address or phone number changes.

We will write to you five weeks before your appointment is due, and ask you to contact us. We will then arrange a convenient date for you to see the consultant, or a member of his or her team.

Should your condition worsen while you are waiting for your appointment, please inform your GP.

If you have any questions please phone us on 0123 456 789. You can phone between 8am and 8pm Monday to Friday. Outside these times, you can leave a message on our answerphone. Please leave your name, hospital reference number (found at the top of this letter) and daytime number, and we will phone you back the next working day.

Yours sincerely

First invitation to telephone

Dear

You can now arrange an appointment with

Consultant's Name and Specialty

by phoning the appointments office on 0123 456 789 to agree a date and time.

You can phone between 8am and 8pm Monday to Friday. Outside these times, you can leave a message on our answerphone. Please leave your name, hospital reference number (found at the top of this letter) and daytime phone number, and we will phone you back the next working day.

If you no longer need to make an appointment please let us know.

If you have any questions please phone us as soon as possible on 0123 456 789.

Yours sincerely

Reminder letter sent when patient has not responded.

Dear

We recently asked you to make an appointment to see

Consultant's Name and specialty

You have not yet arranged to do so. Please contact the appointment office on

0123 456 789 to arrange your appointment.

If you no longer need to make an appointment please let us know.

You can contact the appointment office between 8am and 8pm Monday to Friday.

Outside these times, you can leave a message on our answerphone. Please leave

your daytime number, and we will phone you back the next working day.

If you do not contact us within 2 weeks of receiving this letter, we will assume

that you no longer need your appointment. You will be removed from the waiting

list. We will also let your doctor know that you no longer need your appointment.

If you have any questions please contact the appointment office.

Yours sincerely

Letter to patient advising of removal from the Outpatient Waiting List

Dear

We recently asked you to make an appointment to see

Consultant's Name and specialty

As you have not contacted us to make your appointment we have assumed that you don't need your appointment. We have now removed your name from the waiting list.

We have also let your doctor know that you have decided not to see the consultant.

If you have any questions please phone the appointment office on 0123 456 789.

Yours sincerely

Letter to GP advising of patient's removal from the Outpatient Waiting List

Dear Dr

You referred

Patient Name, Address, NHS Number, CRN

to **Consultant Name and Specialty.**

We have written to your patient twice over the last 4 weeks to ask them to telephone the appointment clerk to make an appointment.

They have not responded and have therefore been removed from the outpatient waiting list.

If you have concerns about your patient not being seen, please contact your patient and then, if necessary, the appointment clerk on 0123 456 789.

The patient can then be reinstated on the waiting list at their original position.

Yours sincerely

Appointment acknowledgement letter (sent after phone booking made)

Dear

Recently you phoned the appointment centre to make an appointment to see
Consultant's Name and Specialty.
As we agreed on the phone, an appointment has been made for you on **date**
day at **time**
This appointment will be at
location
Enclosed with this letter is a map showing you how to get to the appointment, and indicating parking and public transport stops.
Also with this letter is an information sheet that you should read before you come to the hospital. It tells you important information about the clinic you are going to attend.
If for any reason at all you are not going to be able to attend your appointment, please phone us on 0123 456 789. This will allow us to offer your original appointment to some-one else. We will be able to arrange another date and time while you are on the phone.
If you have any questions please phone us on 0123 456 789. You can phone between 8am and 8pm Monday to Friday.
Yours sincerely

Partial booking letter for pre-operative assessment (sent when patient is to be brought in for assessment)

Dear
You have been on the waiting list for
Consultant's Name and Specialty.
We are now able to offer you an appointment to have your surgery.
Before we can arrange your surgery we need to see you in a pre-operative assessment clinic. This clinic allows us to check your general health and fitness for surgery, and it will also give you a chance to discuss your operation with staff. You will also have the opportunity to book a convenient date and time for your surgery at this appointment.
Also with this letter is an information sheet that you should read before you come to the hospital. It tells you important information about your surgery.
Please phone our appointment office on 0123 456 789 and arrange a convenient date and time for your appointment. You can phone between 8am and 8pm Monday to Friday.
If you no longer wish to have your surgery please phone us and let us know.
If you have any questions please phone us as soon as possible on 0123 456 789.
Yours sincerely

It is evident that the efficient and effective use of theatres are essential to the provision of good and timely patient care. Too often patients are booked for admission on times or dates that they cannot attend, their surgery is cancelled at the last minute, or they are admitted and then found to be unsuitable for surgery.

Preoperative assessment

Figures for the period April to June of 2003 show that out of all the cancelled operations in Wales, 47% were instigated by the patient. 35% of these postponements or cancellations were on the day, or one-day before surgery was due to take place. The main reasons for the surgery not happening, as shown in figure 33, were that the patient did not attend or that the patient cancelled the surgery because the date was inconvenient.

The Modernisation Agency considers that: *"Pre-operative assessment establishes that the patient is fully informed and wishes to undergo the procedure. It ensures that the patient is fit for the surgery and anaesthetic. It minimises the risk of late cancellations by ensuring that all essential resources and discharge requirements are identified"*[1]

Trusts that have effective and timely preoperative assessment have a lower cancellation rate.

The NLIAH recommends that preoperative assessment should be carried out not more than six weeks before the anticipated date of surgery but not so close that organising another patient (in the event of the first patient being unfit) is difficult. It is advisable to have a list of patients who are willing to attend at short notice. The patient's assessment should not only evaluate suitability for surgery but should also take into account suitability for anaesthetic, understanding of what the procedure and its aftercare entails. Planning for discharge and any follow-up social care can also be discussed and instigated and the opportunity taken for a proper discussion with the patient to ensure

FIGURE 33
Example of trust theatre
utilisation report

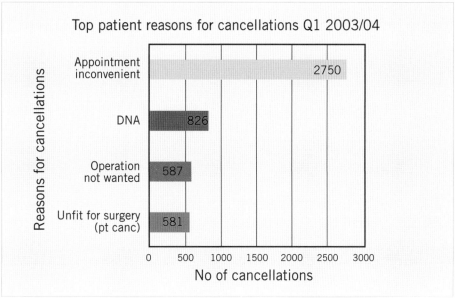

1 *National Good Practice Guidance on Pre-operative Assessment for Inpatients* Modernisation Agency, 2003

Preoperative assessment should be undertaken six weeks prior to surgery, and should be booked using partial booking. Preoperative assessment allows both staff and patient to check suitability for anaesthetic and surgery, agree the booking date for surgery, and organise discharge arrangements

properly informed consent. The consent form can be signed at this point with the patient confirming their decision to proceed when they are admitted. At preoperative assessment, if the patient meets all relevant criteria, negotiation regarding date and time of admission within recognised constraints can take place, and a firm date for surgery can be agreed. This model is part of the booking process recommended by the NLIAH and described on page 71.

The Audit Commission in Wales Acute Hospital Portfolio report[1] states that booking patients before preoperative assessment is common in most Trusts in Wales, as shown by figures 34 and 35. Booking patients and informing them of their date of surgery before determining if they are suitable is one reason for the high number of cancellations, and should be avoided by using the booking methodology described in chapter 3.3. A detailed flowchart of the process is shown in figure 36 on pages 84-85. Pre-operative assessment guidance can also be found in the theatre step guide available at www.portal.modern.nhs.uk/sites/crosscutting/access/Access%20Document %20Library/1/Theatres/Step%20Guide/Complete%20Step%20Guide.pdf

FIGURE 34A
Pre-assessment,
speciality A

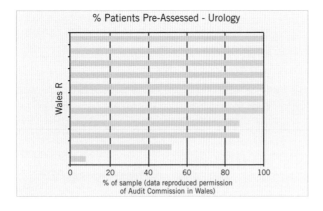

FIGURE 34B
Pre-assessment before
booking, speciality A

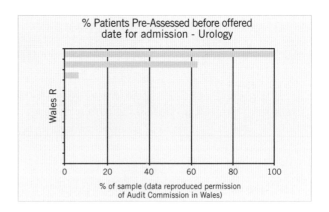

FIGURE 35A
Pre-assessment,
speciality B

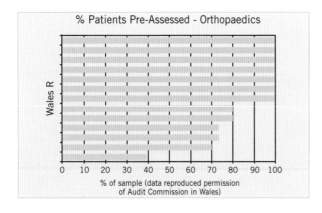

FIGURE 35B
Pre-assessment before
booking, speciality B

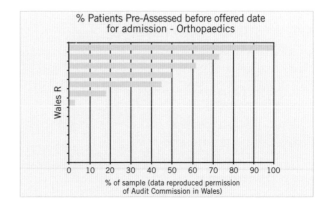

1 *Acute Hospital Portfolio, October 2001, No2* Audit Commission 2001 in Wales

National guidelines for effective preoperative assessment

The National Institute for Clinical Excellence (NICE) has issued a clinical guideline on the use of routine preoperative tests in elective (pre-planned) surgery for children and adults. Carrying out lots of preoperative tests can lead to unnecessary delays or cancellation of operations as well as inconvenience and discomfort to patients because of 'false positive' test results. The NICE guideline will ensure that health professionals have clear recommendations about the tests that should and should not be carried out.

The website address to access these guidelines is http://www.nice.org.uk/cat.asp?c=56818

This also links to the directive delivered in WHC (2003) 137 — Better Blood Transfusions that states clinicians should avoid the unnecessary use of donor blood in clinical practice by securing appropriate and cost-effective provision of blood transfusion and alternatives in surgical care. This can be achieved by ensuring that mechanisms are in place for the preoperative assessment of patients for planned surgical procedures.

Effective training to undertake preoperative assessment

A training package for all professionals working in Pre-operative assessment was launched in September 2002. The training package, a CD-ROM and booklet, is an inter-professional, e-based learning tool, produced collaboratively between the National Pre-Operative Assessment Project, the University of Southampton's New Generation Project and the National training group for Pre-operative Assessment.

To obtain a copy of the package please email preop@soton.ac.uk or MA@prolog.uk.com quoting ref. 29999

Further reading can be found in Chapter 10. Issues about booking, preassessment and day surgery can also be found in 'A Guide to Good Practice: Day Surgery in Wales[1]' available from the NLIAH.

CONWY & DENBIGHSHIRE NHS TRUST

Preoperative Assessment Co-ordinator in Surgery

During the development of an Integrated Care Pathway for patients undergoing Day Case Hernia Repair Conwy & Denbighshire NHS Trust developed an evidence based preoperative assessment phase. Following a successful pilot and evaluation the Modernisation Task Group felt it was important to ensure that all patients undergoing surgical procedures had equitable access to this quality service. A Preoperative Assessment Co-ordinator has recently been appointed and their specific remit is to co-ordinate the modernisation of preoperative assessment across all areas of the Trust.

A baseline audit of existing activity across the Trust is currently in progress and is aimed at measuring where different areas are in relation to best practice. The audit is looking at referrals systems, documentation, processes, environment, clerical, administrative and clinical roles.

A training programme for staff involved in preoperative assessment has been developed, led and piloted by one of the Consultant Anaesthetists.

It is hoped to expand upon this and develop this training programme to provide centralised training for all staff involved in pre-operative assessment across the Trust.

The preoperative assessment co-ordinator will play a key role in ensuring that the Trust will have one recognised process and consistent standards for preoperative assessment and should only be undertaken by suitably trained individuals in an environment conducive to patient's needs.

1 *A Guide to Good Practice: Day Surgery in Wales.* Innovations in Care, 2004

FIGURE 36
Flow chart of the pre-
assessment process

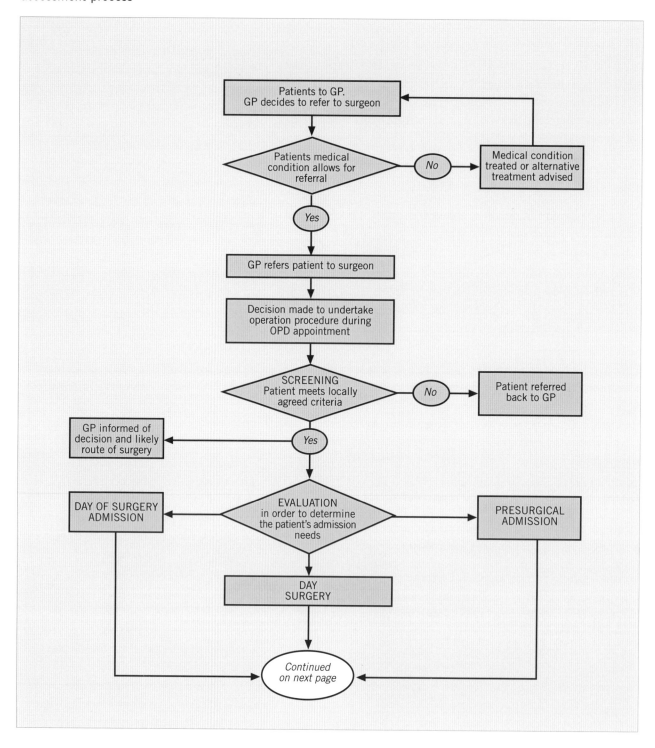

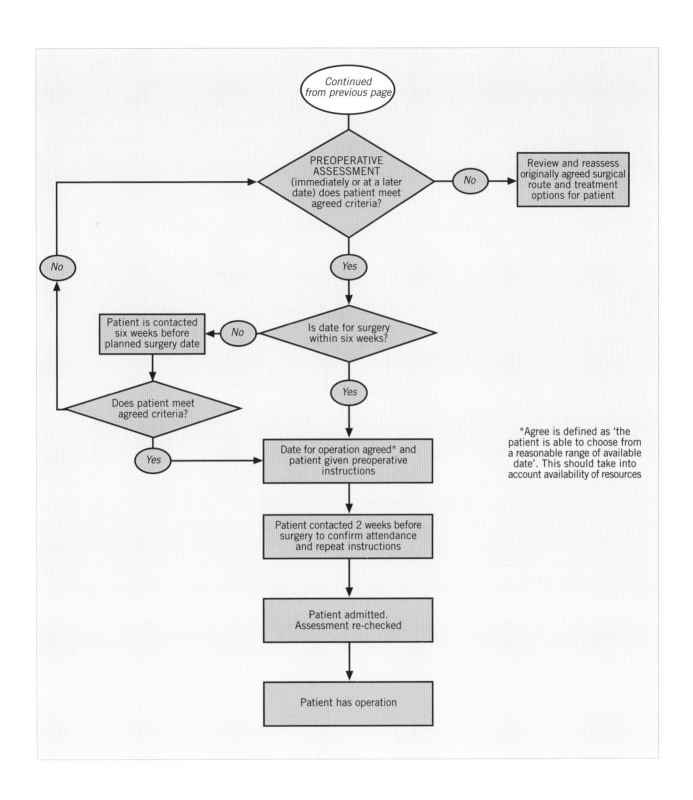

*Agree is defined as 'the patient is able to choose from a reasonable range of available date'. This should take into account availability of resources

Patients are increasingly becoming the focus of all change processes in the NHS. Part 3 of the guide looks at issues around involvement of patients in the change programme.

Key Points

■ Patients must be involved at every stage of the change programme, as a fully integrated and valued member of the team.

■ Effective patient partnerships depend on good communication

■ It is important to have robust strategies in place to find out the views of the patient population

■ Maintaining communication with patients means that patients should receive, as a default, copies of all letters written about their care.

Building Partnerships

Over the last 5 years there has been a political shift towards public involvement in the development and improvement of public services. The recent publication Making the Connections: Delivering Better Services for Wales[1] outlines the importance of putting the citizen centre-stage in the development of all public services.

User engagement or lack of, is one of the main reasons for failure of projects worldwide. Without patient involvement in development of the National Health Service, we may find ourselves with a service which users find difficult to access, to understand and which may not meet their needs. In order for the NHS to function in the modern world, its processes need to be developed to meet the needs of the users.

However, are we all not patients? NHS staff and Community Health Council representatives must have input into the design and development of modern NHS services. But their perspective is shaped by the knowledge of the complex systems and processes through which the NHS operates.

Assumptions may be made based on embedded knowledge of how the NHS functions and the ability to see processes in a fresh light may be limited. Current staff members may be hyper-critical of services, apprehensive of change or make allowances based on perceived limitations of services.

Patient representatives may not have come into contact with these systems before and there is a need to ensure these are designed to meet the needs of ALL patients, without making assumptions of patients' understanding of how the systems work.

Patients' role

The patient's role in service improvement should be as a fully integrated and valued member of the team. There needs to be a joint ownership of the improvement project between the organisation and its patient participant. These patients are not expected to represent ALL patients accessing the services, but to provide a patient perspective on proposed changes and potential improvements. It is vital that a good relationship is developed between the organisation and the patient participants. Staff involved in the project should not see the patient as a threat, but as a professional person working with them to achieve an excellent service in the best interest of all (i.e. staff and patients). Organisations may consider some form of 'bonding' exercise to enable staff to get to know the patients and to give them the opportunity to share feelings and concerns openly so as to clear any misconceptions.

Who wrote this chapter?

This chapter has been written by patient representatives involved with the Implementing the Guide to Good Practice Programme. The patient representatives wanted to demonstrate how they have been able to influence the way services are provided and advise on how to involve patients in improving services within hospital trusts.
A list of the patients involved in the programme appears on the next page.

1 *Making the Connection Delivering Better Service for Wales.* Welsh Assembly Government, 2004

To ensure the above is achieved the Modernisation Agency has developed the Four R's of working together, in its Improvement Leader Guide 'Involving patients and carers'[1] (p16) see figure 38.

A suggested outline of the patient participant's role is as follows. Some of these points may not be covered by the patient participant themselves, but need to be incorporated in the wider organisation's Patient and Public Involvement agenda:

FIGURE 37
The Guide to Good Practice
Patient Partnership Group

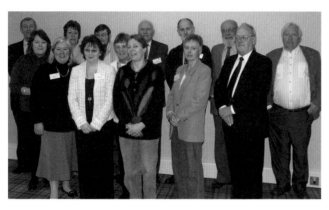

Who we are

A group of people brought together by a common goal — to work in partnership with patients, carers and professionals in order to improve healthcare.

Mr Ken White	*National programme patient representative;*
Mr Alan Oldham	*Powys*
Ms Beryl Davies	*Pembrokeshire and Derwen*
Mr Brian Keith	*North East Wales*
Mrs Christine Roberts	*Pembrokeshire and Derwen*
Ms Christine Pierce	*Conwy & Denbighshire*
Ms Ferenda Driver	*Ceredigion*
Mr Geoff Bell	*Pontypridd and Rhondda*
Ms Irean Morgan	*Swansea*
Mrs Janet Pope	*Velindre*
Mr John Wyatt	*Gwent*
Mr Malcolm Pope	*Velindre*
Ms Mary Cowern	*Carmarthenshire*
Mr Monty Graham MBE	*Powys*
Mr Mostyn Toghill	*North West Wales*
Mrs Nina Weaver	*Gwent*
Ms Pat Carroll	*North West Wales*
Mr Phil Brearly	*North Glamorgan*
Mr Simon Parker	*North West Wales*

■ To contribute to maintaining and continually developing effective public and patient relationships in the organisation.

■ To support, consider and review emerging findings from studies carried out by the organisation.

■ To develop contacts and good working relationships with the range of organisations, patients and communities, which make up the local public.

■ To provide a source of patient views in dealing with particular issues which may arise.

■ To reflect on the experiences of people as patients, service users and carers as well as their wider views of health and social care.

■ To enable the voices of excluded and vulnerable people to be heard and facilitate the involvement of people who are not part of traditional networks and groups.

■ To work in a transparent way in all activities with clear accountability.

■ To participate in other communities if able.

It is desirable that the patient participants should have the following skills:

■ The ability to think creatively and objectively.

■ Good communication skills, including the willingness to contribute thoughts and views for discussion and debate.

■ Effective listening and decision making skills.

■ The ability to work effectively as a member of the team.

1 *Improvement Leaders' Guide: Involving Patients and Carers.* Mordernisation Agency, 2005 page 16

Support, training and induction

As an integrated member of the team, patient participants should undergo similar induction processes as other members of staff. It is the responsibility of the organisation to be open to provide further training and support where identified by the patient and the rest of the project team. Individuals should have a named point of contact to discuss concerns and ideas with.

Patient and staff fears

Patients might be anxious that

- Their views will not be taken seriously
- They will look foolish
- They won't understand what is being talked about
- They may cause offence if they are seen to complain
- It might affect their treatment in the future

Staff might be anxious that

- Their work will be criticised
- There will be unrealistic demands to change services
- Their role and authority might be undermined
- The clinician/patient relationship might be affected
- Patients will lose confidence in them as practitioners if they are seen as vulnerable or not clear

Remit	■ Does the group have clear terms of reference?
	■ Does everyone have a copy?
	■ Has the meaning been discussed so that everyone has the same understanding of what they are they to do?
Role	■ Is each member clear about his/her particular role?
	■ What contribution does each person think they are able to offer?
	■ What do other people think your role is?
Relationships	■ Does each group feel like a working team?
	■ Do people share a common purpose and goals? Have they ever been discussed?
	■ Do you know each other as people, or are you strangers bound by your roles?
Responsibilities	■ What is the group responsible for and to whom?
	■ Is the group clear about issues of responsibility, or is it all left to the chairperson? Does the whole group take responsibility for seeking users views, putting items on the agenda, and ensuring that members have sufficient information for discussions and decisions?
	■ How are decisions implemented?
	■ Is the group clear how decisions that they make are fed into the wider change agenda within the Trust?

FIGURE 38
The four R's of working together

Pontypridd Rhondda CHC were asked if anyone was interested in becoming the patient representative on the Guide to Good Practice project. I expressed interest and had a brief discussion before agreeing to the role. I am particularly interested in initiatives and developments which will improve patient services by doing things differently and by more effective use of technology, better communication between the Trusts and key partners eg. LHBs, Ambulance services, Social Services — and indeed through better internal communication between Directorates and Departments within NHS Trusts. There is a real danger that if we carry on doing the same things, we will continue to get the same results!

I have experience of customer service, the management of change, performance management, and strategic planning, and hope that I can use that experience to ensure that I can represent the interests of patients generally by asking relevant and challenging questions and putting forward sensible and practicable proposals.

Geoff Bell

I was asked if I would like to be a patient panel member for West Cardiff, from that I was asked to join the Innovations in Care Board as a patient representative and have been involved from there with the Guide to Good Practice.
The reasons I got involved are as follows:-
Lay people can sometimes see beyond routines, to try to obtain flexibility and obtain patient feelings in clinical practice.
Best practices in all trusts are shared not for competition but for patients.
To listen to peers and make contribution where I can.
Let NHS practitioners hear patient views and address issues

Ken White

Having recently had the experience of being a patient, there were some things I would have liked to be different. On being invited to join Innovations in Care as a patient representative, I thought it would give me the opportunity to help improve care for others.

Christine Pierce

I am fortunate enough to have recently taken early retirement. I may now be cash poor(er) but the upside is that I am now time rich! My personal experiences of the health service have, to date, been good ones, but I am acutely aware that not everyone is lucky as me. Many people I know are waiting far too long, often in considerable pain and discomfort, before they get the treatment they need.
I hope that by contributing some of my spare time, I can use my experiences as a patient to help to reduce waiting times for everyone. It shouldn't be a matter of 'luck'. We should all receive the best health care it is possible to receive — at the time we need it.

Chris Roberts

Previously being involved with Carmarthen-shire trust for a number of years through my work with Arthritis Care and representing the views of people with disabilities on a patient panel I was only too glad to take things one step further and join the programme.

My driving force behind this work is that patients have a unique perspective of the services they use and are able to offer innovative solutions to service delivery challenges. It is also extremely rewarding as a patient to play a part in this and hopefully make a difference to both the trust and fellow patients.

Mary Cowern

'I have been involved with self management for 5 years, delivering generic Chronic Disease Self Management courses in the community. I became involved with the Expert Patients pilot and was recruited by the LHB onto the IiC Board. I am enjoying being part of an all Wales group. It is exciting being at the cutting edge of change and reform'.

Pat Carroll

Having a positive influence on the changes being made for better patient experience.

Distraction from the less pleasant aspects of life.

I already have community at heart and experience of working as part of a team of volunteers and staff

I want to feel we are doing something worthwhile, helping others to change their lives for the better, helping the community to develop positively.

Mostyn Toghill

I became involved because I have a disabled husband and an elderly mother and I wanted to give something back for all the care they have received from the National Health Service. As a patient myself, I felt I could make a difference by lending any skills and experience I may have to the programme.

I believe very strongly that patients must be involved in decisions made about healthcare. Patients should be regarded as customers or clients, and in order to fulfil customers' needs you must first find out what those needs and expectations are. Patients are a reality check and, I believe, can help to build a better NHS for everybody.

Nina Weaver

I read an advertisement in the local newspaper and telephoned. Then I was invited to the inaugural meeting and having listened to the aims and objectives decided that I might be of some help.

John Wyatt

Rights and responsibilities

Effective patient involvement/participation relies on good communication. It works best when relationships are mature and constructive and when the contribution is sustained over a period of time. The emphasis should be on building partnerships based on mutual trust and respect. The term partnership implies some form of contract (albeit an informal one). The 'contract' between the patient concerned and the organisation requires some basic terms of reference. A contract between two parties presupposes certain rights and responsibilities:

As a patient involved in this project I have the right to:

■ Receive a clear (up front) explanation of the work involved and of the contribution required from me. In the case of a specific project, this should include any formal terms of reference, timescales and outcome measures. Links with other, internal or external projects should be made clear, as should the priority placed on the work by the organisation.

■ Be given an indication of the time commitment required from me.

■ Be introduced, at an early stage, to the other people involved in the work.

■ Be involved from the beginning of a defined project, and at all subsequent stages, including evaluation and/or feedback.

■ Be involved in all discussions regarding the project. It is particularly important that I am involved before minds have been made up regarding the shape and size of the problem — and not just at the stage of identifying and agreeing solutions.

■ Have an identified point of contact within the organisation that will answer my questions and discuss my needs.

■ Receive feedback regarding the quality of my contribution.

■ Receive adequate and timely communication. This to include minutes/notes, agenda and the same briefing documents as the other members of the team.

■ Be given clarity regarding remuneration/expenses including mechanisms for claiming expenses.

■ Have my contribution valued.

Developing a partnership model

Traditional medicine falls into an 'Expert Advisor' model of care. Increasingly, we are moving to a true partnership model to express the relationship between staff and patients:

Expert Advisor	Partnership
Define patients needs	*Elicit patient needs*
Give advice	*Discuss options*
Solve problems	*Explore solutions*
Decide what information they need	*Ask what information they want*
Encourage dependency	*Empower and enable*

As a patient involved in this project I have a responsibility to:

- Be clear and realistic about the time I am able to commit.

- Let the organisation know, in good time, if I am unable to attend meetings and briefings as required or if I am unable to contribute to a previously agreed timescale.

- Accurately share the views, knowledge and experience, which I have gained by using the NHS. While I am in no way required to be a 'universal patient', I will try to ensure that I don't personalise issues but try to reflect as broad and evidence-based a perspective as possible.

- Respect the views of others.

- Maintain my independence. There will be times when I may disagree with managers and staff. At those times I will put my case forcefully and succinctly but, if necessary, I will 'agree to differ'.

- Not allow any personal agenda to influence my contribution or decision-making nor use my role as a patient involved in service re-design to advance my own interests.

- Respect individual and patient confidentiality.

- Deal responsibly with issues of corporate confidentiality[1].

- Strive to work with the NHS and not against it.

- Occasionally, be prepared to 'take the long view' — the NHS is a large and complex organisation and sustained improvements in service delivery can sometimes take time to implement.

[1] Public Interest Disclosure Act 1998

*Patients should be
involved as partners at all
levels of the improvement
process. Patients should
be represented on all
project teams, and
patient views sought on
proposed solutions.
It is not possible to build
a quality service without
an active partnership with
patients.*

*Staff are not a substitute
for patients. Avoid the
easy option of saying that
'all staff are potential
patients'. Staff who are
patients can offer
valuable insights into
problems with services,
but they are not
independent. They will
always carry their
perspective from working
in the NHS, which will
filter their perception of
service delivery, and will
rarely lead to the same
insights as the
independent patient.*

Selection and engaging patient participants

In order to obtain the greatest gains from patient involvement, organisations first need to be clear about what it is they are trying to accomplish before deciding who to involve and how to engage them. Consideration should be given to:

■ Those who have direct experience of the service

■ Members of the wider public

■ Those who represent community interests

Organisations need to be sensitive and consider representation from different socio-economic groups reflecting ethnic, social, cultural and religious backgrounds. Consideration must also be given to those with mental illness, learning difficulties, physical disabilities and all ages to ensure an open, fair and inclusive representation.

Carers also play a key part and in many cases are important advocates for patient's especially when a patients condition or circumstances may affect their ability to speak on their own behalf. They should also be invited to contribute their own perspectives on issues concerning or affecting the patient's experience and can make a vital contribution toward planning, evaluating and improving services.

So how can patients or carers be engaged to become participants? This may seem like an odd question when hundreds of patients pass through Trust doors and use the services of NHS organisations each and every day. However this is a question frequently asked. There are in fact many ways in which to engage patients to become participants and the following list may provide some guidance and new ideas to help.

■ Posters in waiting rooms, clinics, wards and GP practices

■ Advertising on the organisation's website or hospital radio

■ Advertising in local community groups, support groups, leisure centres and libraries

■ Linking with Patient Panels and the Community Health Council who will be able to offer advice about who can help

■ Using clinical staff who have day to day contact with patients to recruit

■ Advertising in local press and on local radio

■ Linking with Expert Patient groups

■ Make use of contacts within local communities such as health care staff and link workers

It is often a good idea to go out and meet with different community groups rather than expecting them to come to meet you. Hold meetings in local community centres, or ask for a slot on the agenda of one of the communities own meetings.

FIGURE 39
Velindre NHS Trust
Patient and Public
Involvement poster

Patient and Public Involvement

 Velindre Cancer Centre / Canolfan Ganser Felindre

Malcolm Pope (Chairman, Patient Liaison Group), Lisa Miller (General Manager)
Velindre NHS Trust, Cardiff, UK

 FELINDRE / VELINDRE

Patient Liaison Group

'The Listening Voice'

A voice for cancer patients and carers in Velindre Cancer Centre

Please address any correspondence to the Chairman, Patient Liaison Group c/o Velindre Cancer Centre

plg@velindre-tr.wales.nhs.uk

Velindre Cancer Centre
Canolfan Ganser Felindre

Objectives

The aims of the Velindre Patient Liaison Group are to:

• Ensure the patient's 'voice' becomes an integral part of the management process.

• To ensure patients, their carers and families are involved in new projects, service changes/modernisation, changes to environment, etc

• Provide a link to the wider group of patients and carers via consultation, complaints and participative involvement.

Background

The Patient Liaison Group was established within Velindre Cancer Centre in Spring 2002. The group includes patients, carers, management and professional staff.

Issues discussed have included new projects, service developments, issues around staff training, complaints, suggestions.

Method

The meetings provide a forum to discuss and obtain input into current and planned services whilst allowing managers a forum to discuss the patient's view on day to day operation issues.

Individuals from the group are on many committees and action groups within the Cancer Centre e.g. Outpatient Quality Group, Innovations in Care Board, Risk Management Committee and the project group for the development of new linear accelerator radiotherapy machine.

Results

The group have developed a suggestion box, information leaflet and a feedback questionnaire [fig. 1].

The group launched an information bag in September 2003. This is now given to all new patients attending the Cancer Centre and Outreach Clinics. The information bag is sponsored by local businesses and is designed to give patients a range of useful pamphlets [fig. 2]

Contents of Information Bag

Guide to local services
Patient Liaison group
I wish I'd asked
Patient guide to local support groups
Hospital map
Ambulance transport
Health eating – your questions answered
The Tenovus Welfare Right Department
Macmillan Cancer Guide
List of Consultants and contact numbers
Questionnaire
Consent – what you have the right to expect
Patient Information Centre

Fig. 2

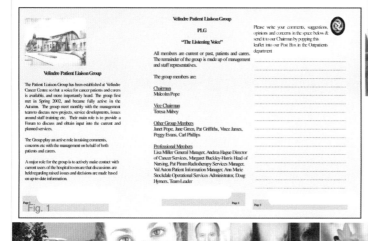

Fig. 1

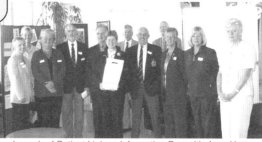

Launch of Patient Liaison Information Bag with Jane Hutt

Conclusion

There has been successful inclusion of members of the Patient Liaison Group in a wide range of strategic and improvement projects, as well as operational issues.

The projects taken forward from the Patient Liaison Group have been actively supported by managerial and professional staff.

Remuneration and Expenses

It is essential that adequate funding is identified and made available to support patient involvement within organisations to ensure commitment from patient participants.

Patient involvement provides an invaluable resource to organisations and many patient participants dedicate a large amount of time and commitment, helping them to improve the services they provide. It is therefore important to be sensitive to financial arrangements for patients as it is inappropriate for them to be the only ones involved who are not being paid. As such, organisations must ensure that patient participants are reimbursed for any reasonable out of pocket expenses incurred whilst fulfilling their role. This may include costs such as mileage, public transport, care costs, stationary and overnight accommodation where needed.

The level and rate of remuneration needs to be discussed and agreed with the individual patient participant at the outset and procedures must be put in place to ensure that their expenses payments are timely. It is important to note however that it may be the decision of the patient participant not to claim the expenses offered, as they may want to provide their services on a voluntary basis.

FIGURE 40
Some key Do's and
Don'ts

Do	*Don't*
■ *Involve patients at every stage*	■ *Use staff members to substitute patient representation*
■ *Ensure roles and responsibilities are clearly defined*	■ *Use jargon in communications*
■ *Provide support, training and induction*	■ *Presume the patient understands all the detailed processes*
■ *Be open and honest*	■ *Be tokenistic about patient involvement*
■ *Be clear about time commitments*	■ *See the patient as a threat*
■ *Be inclusive of all socioeconomic groups*	■ *Assume the patient understands their role at the outset*
■ *Agree remuneration at the outset*	■ *Assume one patient will represent the views of all patients using the service*
■ *Provide clear lines of communication*	
■ *Provide feedback and evaluation*	
■ *Ensure confidentiality*	
■ *Provide a link person within the organisation*	
■ *Involve carers*	

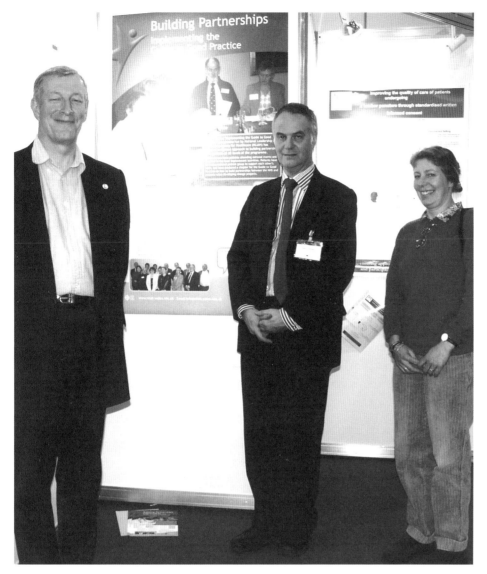

FIGURE 41
Patient group poster at
the 10th European
Conference on Quality
and Safety in Healthcare
April 2005

In some circumstances payment over and above incurred expenses may be
agreed locally between the patient participant and individual organisation.
If this is the case it will be the responsibility of the individual organisation to
discuss and agree the level of payment with the patient participant at the
outset and to ensure that payment is made in line with set procedures for
'Income Tax' and 'National Insurance'.

It is essential that whatever remuneration is agreed that it is made clear to the
patient representative that their commitment and input is valued, that their
involvement is treated seriously and that it will be followed through to achieve
results.

Confidentiality

It is the responsibility of the trust to ensure that patient representatives are
aware of their policy on confidentiality and this can form part of the induction
process. The induction process should also include details and an explanation
on whistle blowing and the difference between this and confidentiality. Patient
representatives should be asked to agree and understand that they will be party
to sensitive discussions that need to be kept out of the public arena.

Communication issues

The communication process with the patient participants should be a two-way process. As the patient is considered an equal member of the team, the same information that is shared to the rest of the team should also go to the patient participant. NHS staff should avoid assuming levels of knowledge and understanding when relaying this information, and during all team meetings. Avoid jargon in papers as well as during meetings, and NHS staff should expect to be questioned over any jargon used in meetings or presentations.

Feedback and evaluation

Feedback and evaluation is an essential requirement for patient representatives and this should occur on a regular and on going basis. Patient representatives give their time free of charge, they need to know therefore that their time is being used valuably. Feedback should include what improvements have been made and whether these are sustainable. If recommendations have not been taken forward the reasons for this need to be explained.

FIGURE 42
A quick check list

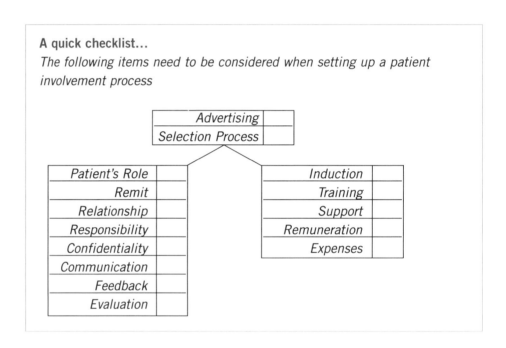

A quick checklist...
The following items need to be considered when setting up a patient involvement process

Advertising	
Selection Process	

Patient's Role		Induction	
Remit		Training	
Relationship		Support	
Responsibility		Remuneration	
Confidentiality		Expenses	
Communication			
Feedback			
Evaluation			

FIGURE 43
Gwent Healthcare NHS
Trust Patient Panel poster

Do you have something to say about your health services?

How about being involved **in planning services** as an important member of our all new...

PATIENTS' PANEL

The panel needs to reflect the diverse nature of communities within Gwent and applications are encouraged from:

- **everyone, regardless of age**
- **those with physical disabilities**
- **black and ethnic minority groups**
- **those requiring to attend with the support of another person**

Your views will help build a better health service in Gwent.

Contact Rhian Lewis at
Gwent Healthcare NHS Trust

By phone: 01633 623812
By e-mail: rhian.lewis@gwent.wales.nhs.uk
By letter: Room 12, Grange House,
Llanfrechfa Grange, Cwmbran NP44 8YN

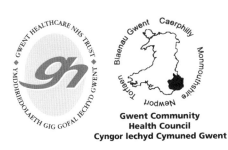

**Gwent Community
Health Council
Cyngor Iechyd Cymuned Gwent**

FIGURE 44
Gwent Healthcare NHS
Trust Patient Panel
recruitment form

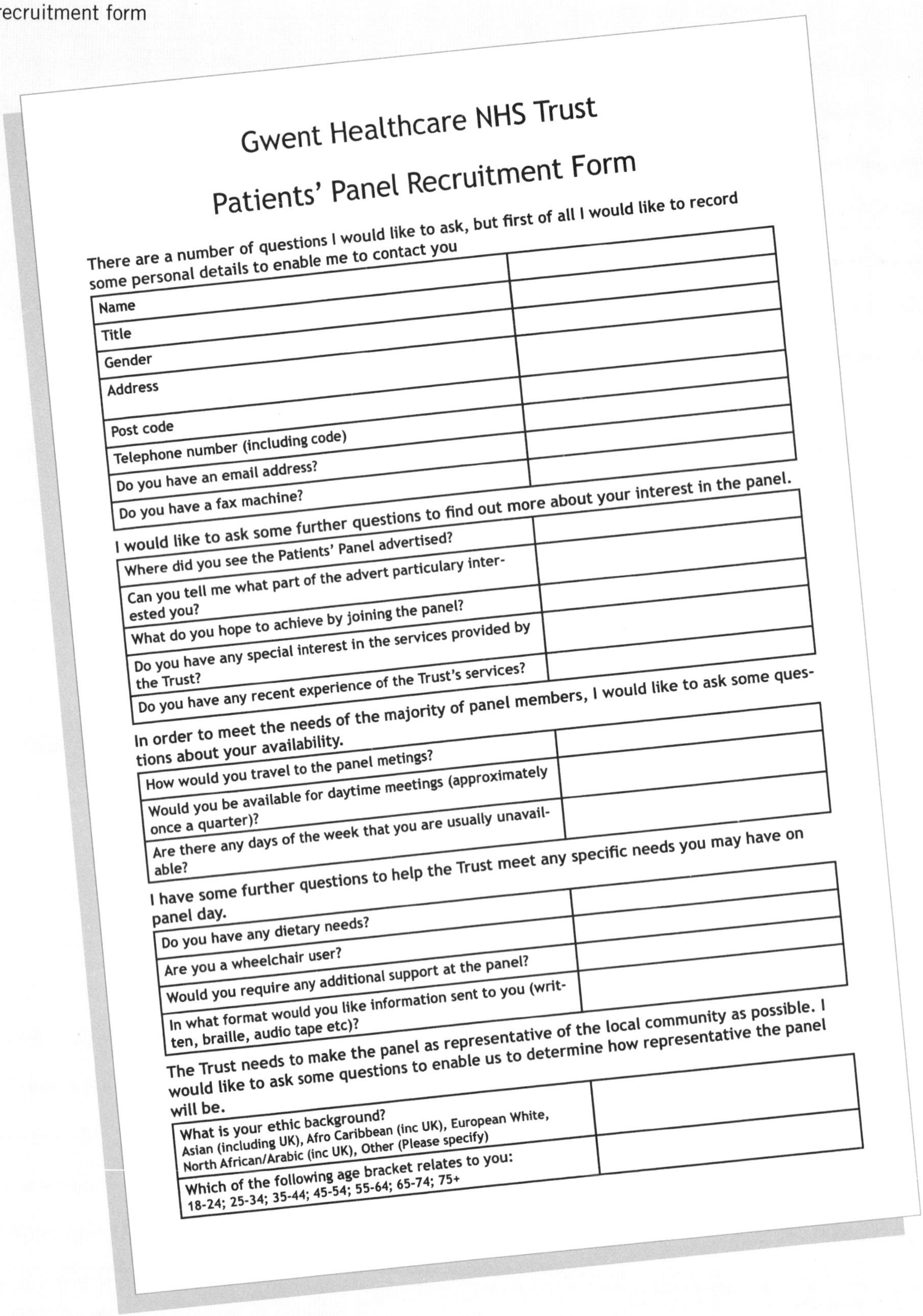

Gwent Healthcare NHS Trust

Patients' Panel Recruitment Form

There are a number of questions I would like to ask, but first of all I would like to record some personal details to enable me to contact you

Name	
Title	
Gender	
Address	
Post code	
Telephone number (including code)	
Do you have an email address?	
Do you have a fax machine?	

I would like to ask some further questions to find out more about your interest in the panel.

Where did you see the Patients' Panel advertised?	
Can you tell me what part of the advert particulary interested you?	
What do you hope to achieve by joining the panel?	
Do you have any special interest in the services provided by the Trust?	
Do you have any recent experience of the Trust's services?	

In order to meet the needs of the majority of panel members, I would like to ask some questions about your availability.

How would you travel to the panel metings?	
Would you be available for daytime meetings (approximately once a quarter)?	
Are there any days of the week that you are usually unavailable?	

I have some further questions to help the Trust meet any specific needs you may have on panel day.

Do you have any dietary needs?	
Are you a wheelchair user?	
Would you require any additional support at the panel?	
In what format would you like information sent to you (written, braille, audio tape etc)?	

The Trust needs to make the panel as representative of the local community as possible. I would like to ask some questions to enable us to determine how representative the panel will be.

What is your ethic background? Asian (including UK), Afro Caribbean (inc UK), European White, North African/Arabic (inc UK), Other (Please specify)	
Which of the following age bracket relates to you: 18-24; 25-34; 35-44; 45-54; 55-64; 65-74; 75+	

Finding out the views of patients

The first part of this chapter has dealt primarily with building partnerships with patients in the redesign process. Equally important is ascertaining the views of as wide a group of patients as possible as part of the redesign process. It is essential that patients are involved in designing all methods of soliciting the views of other patients.

Soliciting the views of patients

Do the patients like the service? Phone or mail surveys, interviews in clinic etc, are valuable to determine what parts of the system still need improving. Patient comments are essential to tailoring the service to their needs.

Too often in the NHS, patient surveys have been used to 'pat ourselves on the back'. The purpose of surveys should not be to find out if the Trust is doing a good job; they should be explicitly aimed at finding out what can be improved. There are a number of tools to help in this process.

Written Surveys

The easiest way to gain information is through the patient survey, and this often elicits the least information. However patient surveys do have a place. Regular surveys of patients can be used as a quick and easy way of keeping a watch on the state of the service, and results collated over time can show up trends.

When designing the survey, it is important to ask first "Why?" The purpose of the survey will help frame the questions, and will affect the method of analysis. Then ask "How will we analyse this survey?" Too often survey forms are designed backwards; a form is created (incorporating all the questions anyone may ever want to know the answer to), circulated and collected. Then someone is asked "How do we analyse this information?"

The design of patient surveys should go through the following sequence of questions:

1 What question is being answered by this survey?

2 What information is needed to answer the question?

3 How will the information be presented once it has been analysed?

4 What sort of analysis will be necessary to allow this form of presentation?

5 What data must be collected, in what format, to allow that analysis to be done?

6 How will the data be collected?

This design process is the reverse of the process the actual data will follow — start at the end point to ensure that everything is in place to allow the process to be completed.

Surveys should be used to monitor positions over time, using graphical output to show trends. They can also be used to solicit a wide number of views quickly. Tick box surveys are quicker to complete and analyse, but solicit a poorer quality of information. Open questions such as "please tell us of any problems you experienced at the reception desk" will give more information than check boxes or questions that elicit a 'Yes/No' answer, but they are harder to design and analyse, and more of a burden for the patient to complete. You should take into account the burden of completing the form, if for no other reason than that you will get better results if the survey is easy and quick to complete.

Most people are not professional survey compilers. When in doubt, talk to your audit department about survey design.

FIGURE 45
North Glamorgan NHS
Trust Patient Focus group
resource pack.

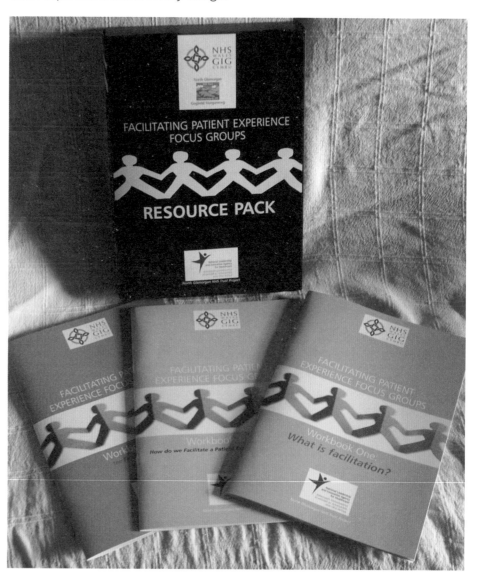

Patient focus groups

Focus groups can also be useful in providing regular feedback on services and in identifying areas that need improvement. Where focus groups are being contemplated, trained facilitators should be consulted and used in designing and running the groups. Questions to be covered by the group should be clear, and time must be given to allow those involved to raise other issues that may concern them. Above all, the focus group should be seen as belonging to the patients, and not to the facilitator or Trust.

Patient diaries

A powerful but time-consuming tool is the use of a patient diary. Asking a patient to record their thoughts and feelings about their care as they pass through the process can be valuable but will be a significant burden on the patient at a time when they may be experiencing stress and vulnerability. Patients must have the process explained to them clearly, be given a choice of written or recorded diaries, and above all it must be clear that they can opt out of the process at any time.

Patient diaries have given greater impetus to change service delivery than any other tool.

Patient walk through

An alternative to the diary, for shorter patient care processes, is the patient walk through. This is typically used as an aid to process mapping, giving a clear view of the process from the patient point of view.

The process involves a member of the improvement team shadowing a patient from the time they arrive at the front of the hospital, to the time that they leave the premises. Everything that happens is recorded using the process mapping approach of 'one person, one place, one time'.

If privacy concerns are met, a valuable aid to the walk through is a camera, so that a photographic record of the patient journey can be compiled. This, coupled with a diary from the patient, can give a more complete understanding of the patient process than any other tool.

Who should do the walk through? Some Trusts have found non-executive directors to be particularly interested in this tool. As well as giving them a better understanding of the processes within the Trust, it will give valuable insight when the improvement projects require Board level decisions.

Copying letters to patients

One area where all organisations in the NHS can improve their partnership with patients is by copying letters to patients.

Enabling patients to receive a copy of letters written about them by one professional to another should be seen as an essential part of good clinical care. It should improve communication between patients and healthcare professionals, and also improve the patient's ability to understand and make choices about their own care and treatment.

This practice is policy in England, and the Welsh Assembly Government is currently undertaking a scoping exercise to determine what form the initiative will take in Wales. Much of the good practice described here is based on the English policy and experience.

Why copy letters to patients?
Overwhelmingly, surveys of patients and carers show that they want to see copies of letters about their care. Evidence is available from England, and some departments in Welsh Trusts, that copying information to patients reduces errors, improves communication, and leads to better standards of care.[1] There is little evidence that patients do not want to see this information.

Copying letters should be the default policy of all NHS organisations, with a clear 'opt out' option explained to patients on their first, and preferably subsequent visits. As a first step, and a minimum standard, patients must be informed of their right to receive copies of all letters, and supported in their requests to receive such copies.

What letters should be copied?
All letters between two health professionals should be included in the copying process. This includes referral letters from GPs to the trust, letters from clinical staff to the GP, and letters from clinical staff to each other. It should also include letters to outside agencies such as Social Services.

Single results, such as laboratory reports, or x-ray reports, should not be copied. The information in these reports is likely to be included in subsequent letters in many cases, and there is consequently no need to copy the raw data to the patient.

Who should receive letters?
Letters should be copied to the patient and their carer where appropriate. The patient must retain the right to receive a copy of their letter, but not have it copied to the carer, if they wish. In the case of children, the letter would go to the carer in most circumstances.

> **GOOD PRACTICE POINT**
> **Copying Letters to Patients**
>
> *All communications between health professionals should be copied to the patient. Patients must be given the right to opt out of receiving letters. Good practice is to write all letters to the patient, and copy the letter to the other health professional.*

1 *Copying letters to patients: Summaries of 12 pilot project sites.* Health Organisations Research Centre, Manchester School of Management, 2003

The Wales Epilepsy Unit at the University Hospital of Wales routinely copies all letters to patients unless there are specific reasons to do otherwise. Diagnoses, management plans, medication and lifestyle advice are also communicated and can thus be read and reread away from the stress and distraction of the clinical environment.

SWANSEA NHS TRUST

The diabetic and lipid clinic at Morriston Hospital copies all letters to patients routinely. Staff consider this process to be essential as a supplement to the advice given verbally to the patient in clinic. Letters also include the results of blood tests and explanations of what the results mean.

The consultant in plastic surgery at Morriston Hospital issues letters directly to patients who have had an augmentation procedure. This is because the consultant feels that some patients may not fully understand what is being said to them in clinic.

In community paediatric services, there is limited routine copying of letters to the parent/guardian relating specifically to the Development Co-ordination Disorder clinic.

There will be explicit situations when it is not appropriate to copy a letter to the patient. Two examples are when the letter contains information about a third party, or when the clinician considers that the letter would be harmful to the patient. In the second situation, the clinician has a responsibility to explain to the patient the reasons why the letter is not sent.

In general, care should be taken to avoid patients learning about bad news by letter, and where a letter contains bad news the patient should receive the letter in an environment where the contents can be explained before the letter is read.

Questions of Jargon

It is often assumed by clinical staff that patients do not need or desire to see letters. As has been stated, the evidence is that the patient view is very different. Another common clinician view is that the patient would not understand the letter if it was sent.

There is some anecdotal evidence to support this belief, although where letters are currently sent, the patients surveyed showed a greater level of understanding than the clinicians had assumed. The solution is to present information in a clear format, avoid the use of jargon, and be explicit in statements made.

There are ways of demystifying letters through the use of substitution (using non-jargon words wherever possible), providing explanations for medical terms in an annex to the letter, or by providing a help line for patients who have difficulty understanding the letters.

A good practice is to write all letters to the patient, and copy the letter to the health professional. This practice, already used by some health professionals, leads to clearer communication and an improvement in the doctor patient relationship.

Translation

In some situations, letters may need to be translated before being sent to patients. Translation can be problematical when technical terms are used.

Experience in England has shown that many patients would be happy to receive their letter copies in English even where this is not their first language.
Where translation is desirable, formatting the letter in such a way that the key points are at the start of the letter and outcomes and actions are at the end, then only translating the key points and summary, is a reasonable compromise.

Where possible, patients should be able to request translations of letters as well as large print versions.

Conclusions

The process of moving towards all patients who want copies receiving them will be a difficult one. There are IT and cost implications, although these may ultimately not prove to be as significant as they may seem at first glance. However, there is no doubt that informed patients are better able to participate in their own care. They are likely to pick up on mistakes and errors that they find in letters thus reducing risk. Above all, patients want to see this information. Twenty years ago patients were not able to see their own medical records. That situation has now changed, and copying letters to patients is the logical next step towards a more open and patient centred health service.

Developments in England

Good practice guidelines 'Copying Letters to Patients' have been issued in England to assist NHS organisations in putting the policy into practice. These guidelines have been informed by the results of pilot studies, which aimed to test key aspects of issues relating to implementation. Copies of the guidelines can be obtained from the Department of Health[1] website.

The way forward in Wales

Close links have been established with the initiative in England. In Wales a number of pilot studies have been conducted in order to test implementation on an organisation wide basis such as a hospital or GP practice. The results of these studies and further developments in England will be used to inform how the copying letters initiative will be taken forward in Wales.

Copying Letters to Patients

An Assembly initiative was piloted at three trusts, to identify whether patients should be sent copies of letters as a matter of course or sent letters subject to specifically requesting them. The pilot proved positive.

CARMARTHENSHIRE NHS TRUST

Some patient feedback "It helps to know that you have been listened to, and that you are both singing from the same hymn sheet", "The consultant explained to me quite well; with the letter it was clearer." "Excellent scheme. It was very interesting to read what the doctor wrote about me and more helpful than what he told me during the consultation", "The letters are a very good idea because at the time of the consultation, some patients may be anxious or simply do not take in or understand what is being said. The letter gives you more to digest and understand".

POWYS LOCAL HEALTH BOARD

When patients did receive copies of their letters it appears from the feedback that they found the experience worthwhile. However, there appears to be less uptake when patients have to request a copy of their letter.

NORTH GLAMORGAN NHS TRUST:

Within respiratory medicine 150 patients were asked if they would like a 'copy letter'. 147 patients responded that they would which is some 98%. Both within respiratory medicine and later in paediatrics, 247 patients who had recently received a 'copy letter' were sent a patient satisfaction questionnaire with six outcome measures. Overall the response rate was 48% which is very good. The results from the patient satisfaction questionnaire were also very promising.

1 *www.doh.gov.uk*

Part 4 of the guide focuses on tools and techniques for understanding the service and for managing projects. The chapters here cover a broad range of issues from basic analysis tools, through project management to Integrated Care Pathways.

Key points
- There are three essential measures that managers must use to understand their services:
  - Process maps
  - Activity, Backlog, Capacity and Demand graphs
  - Flow Models

- Process maps, prepared by teams containing a full cross chapter of staff and patients, are the single most useful tool to understand what goes n in a service

- Capacity and demand analysis, in units of time, are the only way of determining the capacity needs of the service

- Understanding how patients flow through a theatre session or clinic will help improve efficiency and make better use of capacity

- Trend analysis on demand, and an understanding of follow-up demand, will assist planning of services

- Understanding and eliminating carve-out will increase effective capacity

- Central to ongoing performance is a robust set of Key Performance Indicators

- Statistical Process Control is a useful tool to separate the information from the noise

- Traditional methods of managing projects will make them more likely to fail; Critical Chain project management will support project success

- Integrated Care Pathways are one way of introducing consistent methods of work into clinical practice.

Essential measures for managers

5

Staff managing clinical departments need to understand a number of key elements of the services they are responsible for. They must know the capacity of the service, activity levels, and the level of demand on the service; the processes that are involved in the service; and the management of flow around constraints in the system.

Understanding the service: Three essential measures for managers
Managers often talk about capacity and demand for services making assumptions that (a) all their problems are caused by a lack of capacity, and (b) if only the Local Health Board commissioning the service would provide more capacity, they would be able to improve services and reduce waiting times. This is not true.

Commissioning is not the solution. Time after time the requests for more resources are refused, not because the LHB is unwilling to improve services, but because the requests are based on 'more of the same, at the same price' rather than grounded in good information and demonstrated need based on hard information.

Many clinicians and managers do not fully understand the services they work in. There are a number of reasons for this; the NHS is poor in the provision of good information, many managers work in a state of continual 'fire-fighting', clinicians are caught up in an endless progression of overbooked clinics and long waiting lists. There is a way out of this information vacuum.

The National Leadership and Innovation Agency for Healthcare recommends the use of three key pieces of information which will provide the basis for informed process change and performance improvement: measurement of activity, backlog, capacity and demand; process mapping; and patient flow modelling.

The three tools are:

- Process Maps of the key processes in the service;

- Activity, Backlog, Capacity and Demand graphs;

- Flow Models of the use of key constraints in the service.

This chapter deals with these three essential tools.

GOOD PRACTICE POINT

Managing Capacity and Demand

Staff managing services in Trusts must have a clear understanding of the capacity of their service, the activity levels provided by the service, the demand on the service, and the backlog of work in the system. For non-outpatient work some element of casemix must be incorporated into the measures used.

Process mapping

FIGURE 46
The process map

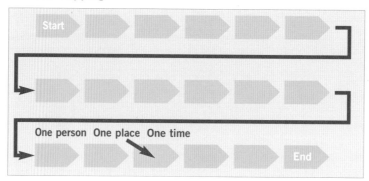

It is important to understand how patients proceed through the service.
The best way to achieve this is through process mapping. Process maps are the ideal way to identify rework within the system, constraints and bottlenecks, and unnecessary process steps. It is unlikely that any one member of staff will fully understand the whole service until the process has been mapped.

Activity, Backlog, Capacity and Demand Graphs — the four measures

FIGURE 47
Activity, Backlog,
Capacity and Demand

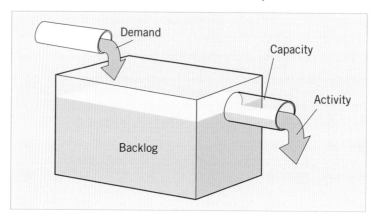

A common unit of measure

Because it is important to compare the four measures on a single graph, the same measures must be used for each. In the example shown in figure 48, minutes of theatre time is used as a common unit, although there are other measures that can be used.

Activity

Activity is the throughput of the system — the number of patients seen in clinic, discharged from the ward, or processed through theatre. The number of patients must be converted to the common unit of measure. Figure 48 shows cataract operations measured in minutes of theatre time.

Backlog

The waiting list needs to be converted to the common measure. The backlog may be the number of patients on the waiting list, or it may be the number of patients refused admission if measuring a process such as bed utilisation. Once again the patient numbers must be converted to the common unit. In figure 48, backlog is represented as the number of minutes of theatre time on the cataract waiting list.

Capacity

The capacity of the system is the time that the resource is available. In the case of theatres, this will be staffed time in theatre. In the case of beds, the total bed nights available. For outpatients, it may be staffed clinic sessions. Capacity is usually measured in time: in figure 48, capacity is surgeon minutes in theatre.

Demand

The demand on the service is all the patients referred into the service from all sources, once again converted to a common measure of time. In figure 48, the referrals are recorded as minutes of theatre time.

FIGURE 48
The combined graph: 4
key measures compared

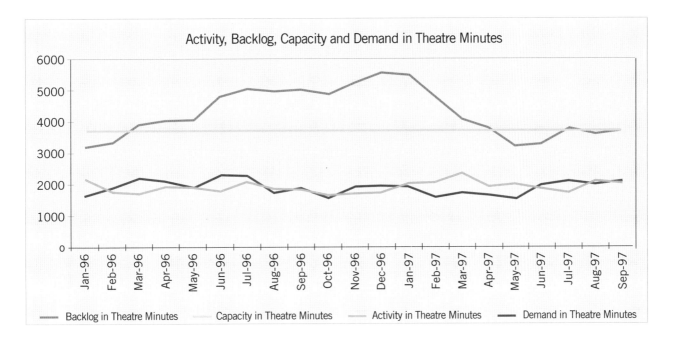

A common graph

Figure 48 shows the four measures for the cataract waiting list, plotted on the same graph. The relationship between the four measures can now be seen clearly. Graphs of the four main measures for key performance indicators should be routinely produced and regularly reviewed.

Flow Models

FIGURE 49
The flow model

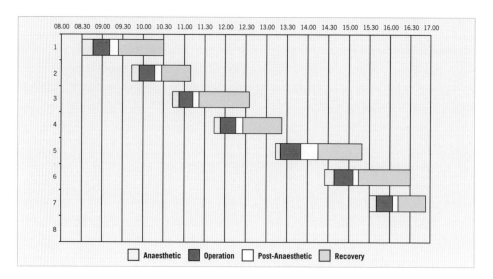

Process maps show the service from the perspective of the patient.
Flow models are a way of analysing the service constraints and bottlenecks found during the mapping process, and looking at them from the perspective of the service.

Flow models are about understanding bottlenecks and determining whether we are scheduling the work around the constraint. In figure 49, the constraint is represented by the red section of each bar. The graph shows that the scheduling of patients in this theatre list is not around the constraint, and there is a large amount of wasted time.

CONWY & DENBIGHSHIRE NHS TRUST
Rapid access nurse led colorectal service

Historically patients presenting with symptoms including rectal bleeding were assessed in the Outpatient department and investigations initiated from that visit. The timing of their outpatient appointment is dependent upon the information provided by General Practitioners and availability of Consultant and appointment slots. From the patient's point of view, a series of visits is often necessary, depending upon the findings of the investigation and the course of treatment.

A nurse practitioner was appointed in October 2002 with the specific objective of improving access to endoscopic diagnostic services. Following successful training and the implementation of agreed protocols and treatment pathways, urgent suspected colorectal cancer patients are seen and diagnosed within 10 working days, reducing the amount of visits to just one.

In addition, the nurse practitioner is able to diagnose and treat common anal conditions such as Haemorrhoids and Anal Fissures. This service involves close and timely follow-up appointments to allow for successful outcomes. The nurse practitioner performs 300 — 350 flexible sigmoidoscopies per annum and 100 — 150 follow-ups.

Enabling nurses to perform such complex and necessary procedures has resulted in a reduction in waiting times for diagnostic services, freeing up the surgical colorectal consultants to see more complex patients in the Outpatient department.

Conclusion
NHS managers do not have the knowledge they need to manage services without an under-standing of and regular monitoring of activity, backlog, capacity, demand and the constraints in the system; the process from the patient perspective and where there are bottlenecks; the flow of work through the service, and an understanding of how to schedule care to make best use of scarce resources.

Process mapping: understanding the whole

Process mapping is ubiquitous in the NHS improvement movement. There is one reason for this: process mapping is the single most useful diagnostic tool for determining where problems lie. Understanding the process from the patient perspective is essential if services are to be improved.

There are two stages to process mapping. First, understand what happens to the patient, where it happens and who is involved. Then examine the process map to determine where there are problems such as multiple hand-offs[1], parts of the process that are unnecessary or do not add value, or parts of the process which would flow better if undertaken in a different order. These problems can be addressed by designing a new more streamlined process.

Second, use process mapping to determine where bottlenecks and constraints occur. Is use of the constraint maximised? Do the patients flow through the system without delays? This approach is covered on page 125 in Chapter 5.4.

Patient processes in healthcare

Patient processes have evolved over time within the NHS with many new systems being bolted on to current processes without an overall analysis of how the whole system functions. There can be many layers to a patient's journey and no one professional has a detailed overview of that journey. It is therefore essential to any improvement work that current systems are mapped by the staff on the ground floor who are directly working within those systems and with the involvement of patients and carers who experience the whole journey from a very different perspective (see Chapter 4: Building Partnerships).

Benefits of process mapping

Process mapping is a very simple exercise, and ensures any improvement work is based on a realistic analysis of current working systems, as opposed to how local policies determine they should be working. It provides a clear indication of where there may be impacts on other parts of the service when changes are made as well as the opportunity to get multi-disciplinary teams from across the healthcare community together to ensure a culture of ownership and continuous improvement is generated. Staff are often not aware of all the complexities involved in a patient's journey and this provides an opportunity for staff to understand how their work impacts on other parts of the system.

The final map itself can be used as a training tool; for communication purposes as well as identifying areas for continuous improvement. The map should be updated when changes are made to ensure current processes are being captured.

1 Hands-off are the places in the patient care process where the patient, or the patient's information, is passed from one member of staff to another. Hands-offs are not only inefficient, they are also a source of clinical error, and should be eliminated wherever possible.

FIGURE 50
The high level process
map

The high level process map

The first step in understanding any service should be to get as many of the staff together as possible, and attempt to map the process at a high level.

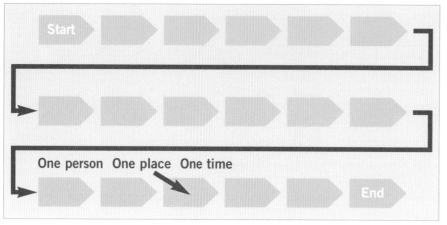

When choosing which patient groups to map try to ensure you are looking at a group who share common characteristics; with high volume for largest impact; where there is a potential to standardise care and a potential for pre-scheduled care.

Choose clearly defined start and end points; for a referral process these may be the arrival of a referral letter in the trust through to the appearance of the patient in the outpatient clinic. For a surgical admission, these may be from the decision to place the patient on a waiting list through to discharge.

The important thing is to be clear which parts of the process are inside the map and which are outside. At this stage a quick mapping exercise by a few staff may be useful to determine who will be involved in a more detailed mapping exercise. It is essential to have representatives of all staffing groups involved in the process at the main mapping exercise, and a quick high level map will help ensure no staff group is forgotten. Do not forget to involve patients in the mapping process.

Organising the mapping event

Once you have a high level process map of the journey you wish to analyse check you have a clear list of all staff groups that are involved in the patient's journey. This will ensure that further down the improvement process when changes are to be implemented, you will already have the staff groups involved on-board and will not have to spend time re-selling the need for improvements to staff groups who have not been involved from the start.

Mapping workshops should be at least a half-day event with all members of staff invited for the whole session, although a drop-in session can be useful where it is impossible to get all staff groups together. In this situation it is vital that all staff involved have an opportunity to validate the final map. If you can get all the staff together there may be time for some action planning at the end of the session, but in any case make sure everyone is aware of the next steps to the improvement process and how they should be involved.

It is advisable to use an independent facilitator to run the event, and it may be useful to run the session off-site, to ensure neutrality. At the outset of the session, ground rules should be set with the group, for example:

■ Freedom for everyone to be open and honest

■ Mapping reality versus what should be happening

■ Focus on what happens 80% of the time

■ Don't make assumptions about people's knowledge

- Clarity over what is being mapped

- 5 minute ruling — if there is debate over a certain step, note the issues and move on after a 5 minute discussion

- The session is looking at processes not people

Throughout the session it may be useful to reiterate some of these rules, and it is essential that there is a blame free culture present. It is a human response to be defensive when groups are looking at the way people work, and the group needs to ensure all staff are focusing on the processes and not the staff involved in those processes.

At the mapping workshop, use 'post-it' notes to capture the information about the patient journey down to the level of 'One person, one place and one time'.

This will ensure that hand-offs, multiple staff, changes in location, and loops in the process are all captured. Capture any issues or suggestions for improvement that are made on a separate flip-chart to circulate with the map when finalised for comments.

Arrange the 'post-its' into order, and look for:

- Things that are done more than once.

- Steps that do not add to the patient outcome — ask "Why is this being done?"

- Count the number of hand-offs.

- Identify where there are delays, queues, and waiting built into the process.

- Ask for each step whether the action is being undertaken by the most appropriate staff member.

- Look for 're-work loops' where activities are taken to correct situations that could be avoided.

It may be useful to re-draw the process map to look at a specific issue. For example, a process map can be drawn with each staff group in a different column to identify the hand-offs — a hand-off occurs each time the process map moves across to a different column.

Focussing in on the problem
Once the overall process map has been drawn and the staff agree with the process, it will be useful to identify where there are bottlenecks in the process.

Which step causes the most delays? This step can then be mapped in more detail, expanding out the process. This can be done several times, each time expanding and getting to a greater level of detail.

FIGURE 51
Looking for hands-offs

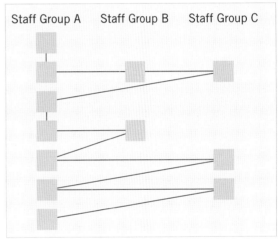

Staff Group A   Staff Group B   Staff Group C

FIGURE 52
Focussing down on the detail

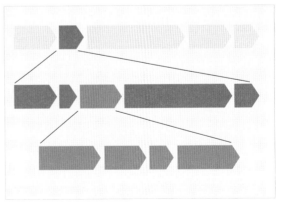

An example might be a map of the cataract process. Initially map the whole process from referral to discharge, with each step representing a hospital encounter. Then focus in on the step with the longest waiting list — maybe the surgical admission. Finally focus down to what happens in theatre.

Any level of mapping is useful, and it is rare for a group to undertake process mapping without identifying at least one step that some members of staff were unaware of. Process mapping is basic and simple — the best way to learn it is to do it.

Some simple tips:

■ Try photographing key steps of the process and illustrating the map for a staff presentation;

■ Walk through the process with a patient to check that all events are included;

■ Work to the 80% rule — there will be differences in the process for different patients — draw the map for the majority;

■ Involve everyone — remember, the porter probably has a better idea than the surgeon where the delays are in the process.

■ Don't forget to include the patient.

Next steps:
Process mapping is the first stage, helping to identify where to start making improvements. The use of Plan Do Study Act (PDSA) cycles of improvement provide a structured approach and framework for developing, testing and implementing changes (chapter 9.4). When looking for potential areas for improvement look for the following:

■ Co-ordinate the patient process of care — promote links throughout the healthcare community

■ Reduce the number of hand-offs and steps within the process

■ Co-ordinate the scheduling of appointments for patients with multiple providers

■ Provide patients with a clear comprehensive care plan at an early stage

■ Create trigger systems so that booking diagnostic tests triggers an appointment for results etc

■ Reduce the number of times a patient has to attend hospital or surgery

■ Reduce or eliminate batching

■ Reduce the number of queues to be managed

■ Extend staff roles encouraging flexibility

Activity, backlog, capacity and demand

An understanding of the dynamics of waiting lists is essential to managing them. There are four key measures that must be understood and monitored on a continuous basis if waiting lists are to be managed effectively. In addition, it is vital to understand the two key types of limitations in the system: constraints and bottlenecks.

Consider the following scenario: waiting lists are increasing, and it is necessary that they are reduced. The demand is 5000 patients per annum, and only 4500 patients are seen in clinic. Waiting lists are going up by 500 patients per annum. What should be done? The Trust asks the commissioning body to pay for an additional 500 cases.

Consider another: there is an increase in waiting times for CT scans. The wait has gone from 12 months to 18 months over the past two years. The data supports the impression that there are more referrals. What should be done? The Trust asks for an additional CT scanner.

Again: waiting times for orthopaedic surgery are over 18 months. The waiting list is increasing. What should be done? The commissioner is asked for an additional orthopaedic surgeon.

There is an unstated assumption behind all three of these scenarios. The consultant in clinic works 100% of the time. The CT scanner is utilised 100% of the time. The surgeon in theatre utilises 100% of the theatre time. These assumptions are usually wrong.

Capacity is the ability to do work, not the amount of work done. It may be true that the CT scanner is working at 100% capacity, but without data for both activity and capacity, two separate and distinct measures, that cannot be assumed.

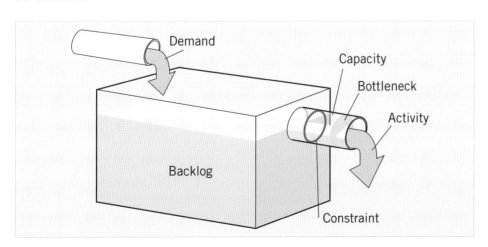

FIGURE 53
The four key measures, and the limiting factors

The NHS collects data on activity, but rarely on capacity. Activity is measured in patient numbers, and is collected for commissioning purposes. There are many systems in place to automate the data collection process. To understand capacity, we need to dig deeper. So what is the relationship between activity and capacity, and how can they be related?

FIGURE 54
What do we mean by theatre availability?

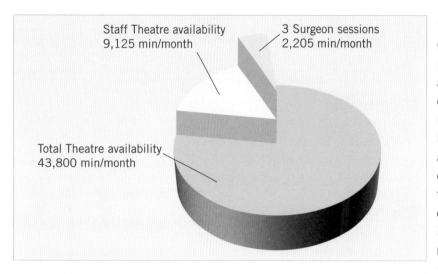

Staff Theatre availability
9,125 min/month

3 Surgeon sessions
2,205 min/month

Total Theatre availability
43,800 min/month

GWENT HEALTHCARE NHS TRUST

Capacity and demand in CT

In August 2002 the Radiology Directorate applied the capacity and demand framework to CT services. There were long outpatient waiting times and it was difficult to balance the priorities of ward patients and urgent outpatients. There was a perception that there was insufficient capacity to meet demand.

The data for a two-week period showed that there was enough capacity to meet current demand but not to address the waiting list backlog.

The process maps indicated a number of tasks to be undertaken and regular monthly meetings were introduced at one site. Some of the improvements to date are:-

- *An increase in the average number of patients seen per session from 10 to 13;*
- *Improvement in timeliness of vetting of referrals;*
- *Delegation of some vetting from Consultant Radiologists to radiographers resulting in less delay;*
- *Reduction in out patient waiting times from around 12 to 8 weeks partly by re-directing referrals to another DGH within the Trust;*
- *Scheduling ward patients at the beginning of each session to make it easier for Consultants to provide reports to clinicians on the same day;*
- *Freed up radiographer clinical time by moving scheduling to clerical staff;*
- *Improved attendance at the evening clinics by over booking to allow for DNA's;*
- *Introduced additional Monday morning session to treat more ward patients;*
- *Developed booking template for all sessions;*
- *Re-organised porter support for the department.*

Measuring capacity

Capacity is the resource available, multiplied by the time it is available. The capacity of an operating theatre is not the number of patients operated on, but the time the theatre is available to be used. Because an operating theatre is 'hardware', the annual capacity of an operating theatre is theoretically 525,600 minutes (43,800 per month). This assumes the theatre to be available for use 365 days a year, 24 hours a day. But theatres must be staffed to be of use. A single shift (7 hours per day, 5 days a week) would give a monthly capacity of only 9,125 minutes, substantially less.

What about the surgeon? For a given waiting list, surgical capacity must be reduced even further. A typical calculation is that a surgeon works 42 weeks each year, so the actual average monthly availability must reflect that reduction. It must also take into account the number of lists (hours) each week that the surgeon spends in theatre. Typically, three half day lists would give a surgeon a monthly theatre capacity of 2,205 minutes.

There are two key points here. Does theatre capacity mean physical capacity? Staffed capacity? Surgeon capacity? And capacity is measured in units of *time*, because the important information is the *time the resource is available.*

Measuring activity

It is not possible to compare two items measured in different units, so if the intent is to compare activity to capacity, activity must be measured in time as well. In the case of outpatient activity, this is relatively simple — assumptions are made about how long it takes to see each patient (usually longer for new patients than follow-ups) and the number of new and follow-up patients attending are multiplied by those times. For theatre lists, diagnostic tests, or inpatient procedures, other measures are necessary. The relative merits of various measures are covered later, but on a basic level, calculate an estimated time for each procedure, and use that time rather than patient numbers when calculating activity. Activity is measured as the total number of patients processed, multiplied by the time it took to process each patient.

Measuring Demand

In order to compare capacity and activity to demand, it must also be converted to time. Demand must be measured by the number of patients added to the waiting list, multiplied by the time each patient is likely to take having the appropriate procedure. Demand should be measured by the additions to the waiting list each day, as historical demand may not show patients added and then quickly removed (for example, acute theatre cases which will affect throughput, and appear in activity data, but may not appear on the waiting list).

It is also essential to ensure that total demand is measured — in outpatients, demand will include GP phone-in patients, or patients sent up from A&E, not just the 'paper GP referrals'. And remember — each patient is converted to time.

Measuring Backlog

The waiting list is also measured in terms of time. Converting waiting lists to theatre minutes is not difficult. Estimated times for each procedure can usually be obtained — in the case of theatres, this data is usually captured in the theatre IT system. The appropriate time can then be allocated to each patient on the waiting list, and the total waiting lists expressed in theatre minutes can be captured at the end of each month. Be careful not to use the average theatre time — see the end of this chapter for the best way to calculate estimated times.

FIGURE 55
The standard presentation
of the 4 measures

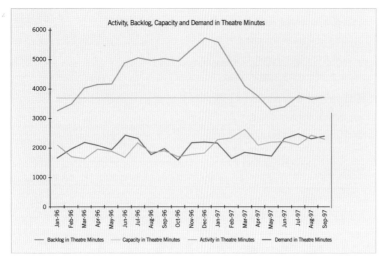

Waiting list in patient
numbers, including trend

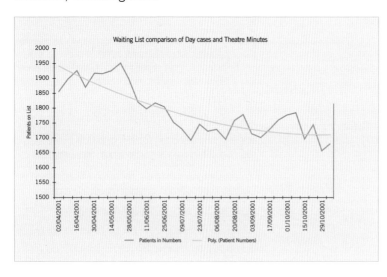

Waiting times in patient
numbers and theatre
minutes

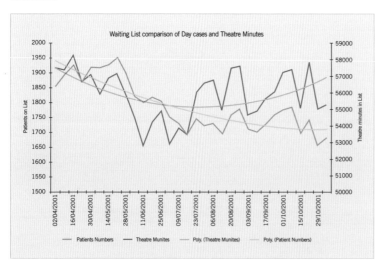

The common graph
Figure 55 shows the four measures for one such list, plotted on the same graph. The relationship between the four measures can now be seen.

Why theatre minutes?
Figure 56 shows the dangers of not using time as a measure. Figure 56A is a graph showing the number of patients on a day surgery waiting list, expressed as patient numbers (or FCEs). The curved line represents a trend for the waiting list, and it can be seen that the trend is down but levelling off. The data line shows a drop over the first part of the graph, with a levelling off towards the end. Clearly, the waiting list has reduced and is under control.

Figure 56b tells a different story. On this graph, the waiting list converted to theatre minutes is superimposed on the original. The trend now looks somewhat different. After hitting a low point part way through the year, the waiting list has started to rise again. It is not under control. Which is correct? Why are they different?

Waiting list numbers measured by patient numbers leave open the possibility of searching the list for short (easy, cheap) cases as a way of reducing quickly the number on the waiting list. The result of this practice is to increase the weight of the casemix of the remaining patients — the casemix on the waiting list becomes steadily more time consuming as the easy cases are selectively removed. The ability to identify easy work, as a way of keeping lists low, is reduced. Ultimately, a point will be reached when the patient numbers will rise rapidly, because the remaining cases on the waiting list are all time consuming ones.

What measures should be used?

The examples so far use theatre minutes as a measure. This is a useful measure for surgery, where theatre time is likely to be the most expensive and scarce resource, but other measures are more appropriate in other situations.

Bed nights

Bed nights, measuring length of stay, is useful for medical patients and situations where there are bed shortages.
For activity, measure actual bed nights; for capacity, number of bed nights in the time period; for demand, the estimated length of stay for those patients booked. Backlog is measured by the estimated length of stay for those patients whose operations were cancelled.

Diagnostic machine use

For equipment like ultrasound, CT, MRI and endoscopy, session time and procedure time make useful measures. Remember that as with theatre time, the equipment is not useful unless the operator is also available, so capacity is the number of operator hours, not the 24/7 equipment availability.

Clinics

Outpatient clinics and therapy clinics should be measured as resourced clinic time. Where courses of treatment are involved such as a planned series of physiotherapy appointments, these are part of the demand on resources, and should not be overlooked.

Case weights

Case weights are useful measures of resource use, as they give a relative value to patients on the waiting list that is more meaningful than the traditional NHS measure of patient discharges (see box).

Case weights are not ideal for improvement work because they are not specific enough in how a particular case weight is derived – for example a short LOS condition with a high theatre component may have a similar case weight to a condition with a long LOS and no theatre component.

Cash

There is one other measure that people use to measure relative worth, and that is cash value. In many respects cash is the same as case weights as a measure for improvement, although it does have the added advantage of showing the actual value of time saved or resource used. The NHS is poor at realising the financial impact of change (or lack of change). Measuring improvement as money saved can be a powerful argument when dealing with commissioning groups.

Constraints and Bottlenecks

Figure 53 on page 117 contains two other items it is necessary to understand in order to manage capacity and demand: constraints and bottlenecks.

In some countries, all resource allocation and commissioning is done on the basis of case weights. The case weight unit is a measure of resource use, and takes into account factors such as length of stay, drug costs, theatre costs, ICU costs etc. averaged for a DRG (Diagnostic Related Group) or HRG (Health Related Group). Commissioning is then done as a number of 'Case Weight Units' for a speciality, sometimes broken down into emergency and elective case weights. The number of patients able to be treated depends on the complexity, and thus the case weights, of their coded condition.
Thus a LTA of 100 case weights may mean that the Trust treats 200 simple (0.5cwu) cases, 25 complex (4cwu) cases, or any combination of cases that add up to 100 cwu.
Commissioning in Case Weight Units gets Trusts and LHBs away from the problems outlined in this guide, of all cases being treated equally, for example the assumption that a total hip revision is equivalent, in commissioning terms, to a carpal tunnel release.

Constraints

The constraint in the system is the factor that ultimately restricts the capacity of the system. In theatres, the constraint may be the surgeon operating on the patient. In outpatients, the constraint may be space. In diagnostics the constraint may be skilled staff to undertake procedures. In every process there will be a constraint which ultimately limits the throughput of the system. The constraint is not easily removed without substantial investment in terms of staffing, or facilities. Identification of the constraint is an essential part of understanding a service.

Once identified, the constraint should become the most important part of the process. Work should be scheduled so that the maximum use is made of the constraint. Resources at the constraint should not be used for jobs that other staff could do. It is poor management to have surgeons fetching their own patients — especially if the reason is to save money on porters!

Bottlenecks

The bottleneck is altogether a different beast. Health processes are complex and full of bottlenecks. A typical bottleneck in theatres may be portering staff — the entire theatre system stops while waiting for a patient to arrive from the ward because of a shortage of porters. Constraints cannot be removed without investment; bottlenecks are usually cheap or even free to remove.

Distinguishing between the constraint in the system and the bottleneck currently limiting activity is essential. Constraints limit capacity — bottlenecks limit activity. By removing bottlenecks it is possible to increase activity until it gets close to the capacity of the system — which the commissioner is ultimately paying for.

Constraints and bottlenecks: a three step process

1 Identify the constraint in the system. Use process mapping (page 113) to determine where the constraints are.

2 Determine whether the process is scheduled around the constraint. Use patient flow modelling (page 125) to determine this.

3 If not, use PDSA cycles to eliminate a bottleneck (page 203) and then repeat step 2.

4 When you reach the point where the use of the constraint is maximised, analyse your capacity to determine whether it is sufficient. If it is not, then it is time to meet with the commissioning group — but now you have hard data.

Maximising use of the constraint: The 80% rule

When calculating throughput do not use averages. Averages are seductive; using the average theatre time to calculate theatre minutes on the waiting list may seem like an obvious solution, but it will usually under estimate the actual demand.

Variation is a normal part of all processes and clinical processes are no different. Accounting for the variation is important when doing the calculations in this section, and averages hide variation. Rather than using the average (50th percentile) you should use the 80th percentile.

FIGURE 57
Average vs 80th
percentile

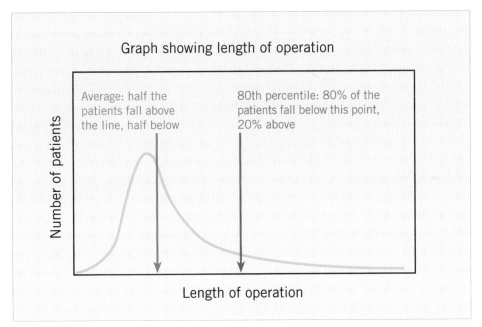

Take 100 patients who have cataract surgery. The average (the median in this case) length of the procedure can be found by sorting the patients by length of procedure, then counting to the middle (patient 50) and seeing how long their operation took. If this figure is used, half the time the operation will take longer than you have allowed, and you will be in danger of running short of time if several patients take longer than average (which they will, 50% of the time). Variation will average out over a long period, but will not average out over a small number of cases such as a theatre list. This is the same issue seen in booking cancer waits (page 67) and described under carve out (page 141).

By counting up to the 80th patient (80th percentile) and using that time, then you are likely to have underestimated the time needed on only 20% of occasions. It is far less likely that you will have a run of patients over the estimate.

Managing patient flow

Process Mapping looks at the care process from a patient perspective. There is another tool that will help identify where the bottlenecks in the process are and how to maximise use of the constraint in the system. Patient flow models look at the care process from a clinical unit perspective, bringing together a number of patient process maps to look at work flows through the unit.

Flow models are the best way to analyse the work of a unit, such as an endoscopy suite, an outpatient clinic, or an operating theatre. The process of building up the model is simple if all the steps are followed.

FIGURE 58
Initial process map

1. Map and agree the process
The process must be mapped to a high level of detail.
A detailed map of theatre may cover the process from the arrival of the patient in theatre until discharge from recovery — each step involving one staff member should be distinct. (Figure 58).

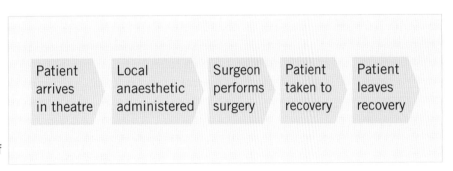

Patient arrives in theatre → Local anaesthetic administered → Surgeon performs surgery → Patient taken to recovery → Patient leaves recovery

2. Time the steps
For a session, record the times for each step of the process. (Figure 59).

3. Identify the constraint
The constraint is that part of the process which is the ultimate restriction on the amount of work that can be done. It is the part of the process that cannot have resources added to improve throughput — it is often the most expensive part of the process. In theatres, the constraint will nearly always be a surgeon operating on a patient. In outpatients, it may be a clinic room in use by a consultant. In an endoscopy suite, it may be a 'scoper' examining a patient.

4. Draw the flow model
Using graph paper, or a spreadsheet programme, draw each patient as a horizontal bar one above the other. Set the horizontal axis to represent time, with the start of the session on the left, and the end on the right. Colour each stage of the process a different colour — it may help to colour the constraining process red. The length of each line will now represent the time each step of the process takes, and multiple patients will show as a series of horizontal lines (see figure 60). Add up the total of the red sections, and calculate it as a proportion of the total time.

In this example, there were seven patients operated on. The total time in theatre (excluding the time in recovery) was 7hr 42min (from 0830 to 1612). The total time a patient was being operated on was 2hr 56min (the total length of the red bars) or 38% of the total theatre time.

FIGURE 59
The flow data

Patient	Start of anaesthetic	Knife to skin time	Operation end time	Patient goes to recovery	Patient leaves recovery
1	08:30	08:45	09:12	09:23	10:30
2	09:43	09:53	10:17	10:26	11:10
3	10:44	10:52	11:13	11:21	12:35
4	11:45	11:52	12:15	12:25	13:20
5	13:15	13:21	13:51	14:14	15:18
6	14:27	14:39	15:05	15:13	16:15
7	15:30	15:38	16:03	16:12	16:53

5. Ask Why...

Over the course of the theatre day, operations took up 38% of the available time (actually even less, because the session ended 18 minutes early). This is not a good utilisation of a very expensive resource. Why are there long periods when there is no surgery taking place? What else is happening during this time? In one case, the delays were caused by the surgeon leaving the theatre to fetch the next patient from the preoperative lounge — because the theatre management had 'saved money' by reducing the number of porters.

FIGURE 60
Actual flow utilisation

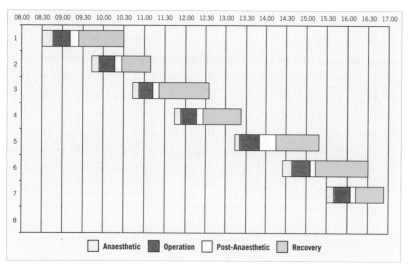

6. Ask How...

How can the situation be improved? It should be possible to schedule the theatre in such a way so as to maximise the use of the scarce resource, which is a consultant operating on a patient. What is currently being done in theatre that could be done elsewhere? Can tasks be undertaken in parallel?

7. What is possible?

It is possible to put together an 'ideal' flow model scheduling around the constraint. Use estimated time for each stage based on the 80th percentile time for each step of the process. This will make it possible to estimate the optimum use of the constraint and give a target to the improvement project. Figure 61 shows that should be possible to double the number of operations.

FIGURE 61
The 'ideal' flow

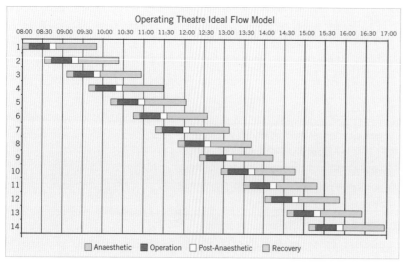

Conclusion

This analysis tool will not show what should be done, or even what the causes of the delays are. Process mapping will provide that information. The tool will show how well scarce resources are used, and how much room there is for improvement.

Additional analysis tools

6

This chapter covers a number of additional analysis tools and procedures that Trusts have found helpful in managing waiting lists. Access to good information, and understanding the meaning of that information, is essential if the NHS is to manage waiting lists effectively.

These tools should be considered additional to the three essential tools in Chapter 5, (process mapping, activity-backlog-capacity-demand monitoring, flow modeling) which are fundamental to understanding services in the NHS.

Understanding demand
This chapter looks at the relationship of demand to activity and the importance of monitoring demand and analysing changes in demand.

Measuring follow-up demand
Follow-up patients in outpatients are one of the main demands on clinic time. But before reducing demand, it is important to understand it, and measuring follow-up demand for outpatient space is difficult.

Reducing follow-up demand
There are a number of tools to manage and reduce the demand on outpatients created by unnecessary follow-up appointments. A few basic approaches are included here.

Carve out: understanding queues
The NHS sometimes seems to be primarily about queues rather than care. Patient experience is often about waiting, and has been described as long periods of waiting broken by short periods of activity. Understanding the principles behind queue management will reduce queues and improve waiting times.

Key performance indicators: what should we monitor?
Knowing what to look for when monitoring clinic performance is essential to getting performance improvement. The NLIAH recommends the use of a number of different KPIs.

Statistical Process Control
Of the tools available to managers, statistical process control is one of the most useful in a wide variety of applications. From bed use to waiting times, from referral to progress through a care pathway, SPC provides a set of tools to analyse performance.

Team working

Within Bridgend, therapists provided allocated sessions to each of the funded Speech and Language resources based within mainstream primary schools.

The Speech & Language Therapy Service had difficulties with recruitment and retention of therapists. Therapists felt isolated, and if a post became vacant an inequality of service across locations resulted. The service was unable to meet demand.

Additional recurrent funding from the LHB enabled a rotation package to be established. Qualified therapists now work as a team across the targeted resources, up dating assessments, jointly agreeing Speech and Language Therapy targets with school staff and other care-givers and preparing programmes.

Each resourced class has additional support from a Speech and Language Therapy Assistant who is able to follow through on tasks set by the therapist for continued direct work.

The outcome of an Audit questionnaire has shown the benefits of this initiative. Therapists no longer feel they work in isolation and are able to support each other clinically . Each school location has received a therapy package of care based on the needs of the individual children within the current level of funding. The Assistant has provided a vital and continuous link between the school and therapy services.

Understanding demand trends

Understanding the demand for services and how it balances against the activity the system is producing, is fundamental in understanding where waiting lists come from and how to deal with them. This chapter addresses issues of activity levels, changing demand and how to relate one to the other.

Demand and Activity

Many analyses of outpatient problems look at the waiting time, or the number of patients waiting. While these are important measures, they are symptoms of a deeper problem. Understanding this deeper problem is essential to any attempt to address outpatient performance. Absolutely the first information required relates to clinic inflows and outflows.

Figures 62A and 62B show two typical outpatient clinics. The number of referrals for each month is shown (Demand), as is the number of patients seen in clinic (Activity). It is obvious that there is variation in both the demand and in activity. The variation is small, and the difference between demand and activity is also small. On their own these graphs are not particularly meaningful. It is necessary to extract the difference between referral and appointments to see the true impact of a relatively small imbalance.

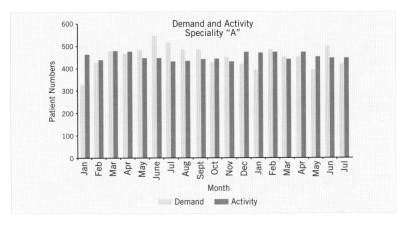

FIGURE 62A
Speciality A demand and activity

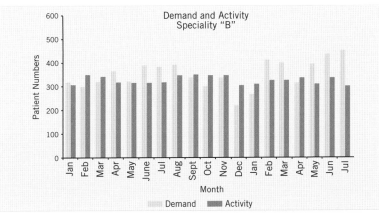

FIGURE 62B
Speciality B demand and activity

Figures 63A and 63B extract that information. The additional line represents the cumulative difference between the inflow and the outflow to the system — the backlog. It can be seen at once that despite significant variations from month to month, the clinic in speciality A is in balance. The variation is around a horizontal line — the backlog remains relatively stable. Figure 63B (Speciality B) tells a different story. There the trend of the line is definitely upward. There are some months where the line dips (possibly due to seasonal variations), but over time, the line creeps up. This speciality is in trouble and the backlog (waiting list) is increasing.

Waiting lists are like water in a bath. As long as the water is running out of the drain as fast as the water is flowing in from the taps, the bath will neither overflow nor empty. The size of the bath doesn't matter — only the rate of the inflow (demand) and outflow (activity). Like the waiting list, the catastrophe occurs when the inflow is greater than the outflow — and the bath overflows.

There are three possible states for any dynamic system such as this. In the first, demand is greater than activity. Over time, waiting lists will increase and waiting times will get longer.

The second possibility is that demand and activity are in balance. This may still not be the ideal situation, because it is possible that the system is in balance, but with a large waiting list of patients in the system. There is a perception that the problem is unmanageable, because there is a huge waiting list — but in fact this situation is far more manageable than the first, because one-off initiatives will have a lasting effect, whereas they will not resolve the first case.

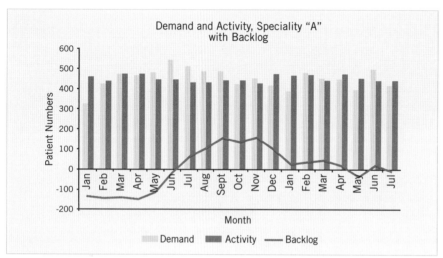

The third possibility is that demand is less than activity. This may seem a better situation to be in (especially if there are large waiting lists) because over time the waiting list will reduce. But as with the slowly draining bath, the situation is no more sustainable in the long term than the first case. In time, the waiting list will disappear, and there will not be enough work to maintain current staffing levels.

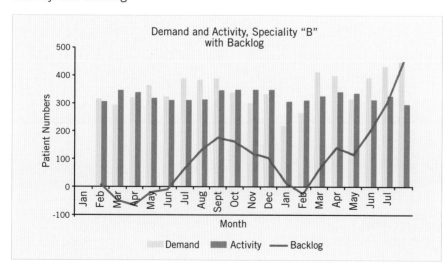

Is it possible to get the system in balance? If a speciality has greater demand than activity, there are only two ways to resolve the problem: permanent increase in activity (one-off initiatives will only delay the day of reckoning) or permanent initiatives to reduce demand. Chapter 9.5 addresses the issue of using feedback to GPs about referrals and this is a good solution to reduce demand. In general, there are many referrals into secondary care that could be handled in ways other than a consultant outpatient appointment, and each of these represents a waste of resources.

Even if the system is in balance, referral guidelines may still be a good idea. The size of the waiting list is in itself a factor in determining referral rates. If waiting times are long, patients will seek other options for treatment and GPs will be less likely to refer. When waiting times reduce (as a result of increased capacity or a one-off initiative) there is less incentive to treat patients, and more incentive to refer into secondary care. Having referral guidelines in place before undertaking the volume reduction initiative will prevent the surge in referrals, and preserve the effect of the extra capacity.

Activity is not capacity

Chapter 5.3 has already dealt with the differences between activity and capacity, and the issues associated with measuring them. Activity is the rate at which patients flow out of the system — off the outpatient waiting list, off the inpatient waiting list. Capacity is only the same as activity when the whole system is operating at 100% efficiency — and experience shows that this is rarely the case. Capacity is the ability to do work. It is a combination of the resources available and the time that those resources can be used.

FIGURE 64A
Trends in referrals,
speciality A

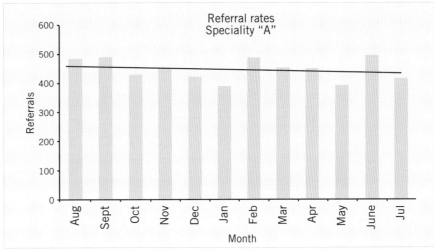

Changes in demand over time
Even if demand is in balance with activity, there is still the risk that it will change over time. Figures 64A and 64B show the number of referrals per month for the past 18 months in two specialities. Figure 64A shows a speciality where the demand is stable or even dropping slowly. It is important to realise that in this case, reducing demand does not mean that there is no problem or waiting list. The speciality may still have an increasing waiting list — because there is less activity than demand.

FIGURE 64B
Trends in referrals,
speciality B

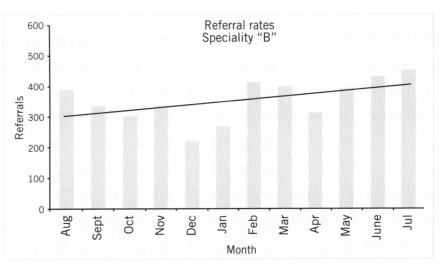

Figure 64B shows a different problem. Since February, the numbers of referrals in this speciality are up on the previous year, despite the seasonal variation. Identifying specialities where the demand is increasing is important in determining what the long term activity will need to be — and how it will need to change over time. Balancing activity and demand today is not going to provide a long term solution because if referral rates continue to increase, the demand will eventually outstrip activity again. The solution is to understand why the demand is increasing, and address that problem.

Seasonal variation

Are referral rates stable across the year? In some clinics, referrals increase at certain times — typically medicine referrals increase in winter, as do those for orthopaedics. Referrals in dermatology increase in summer. Some specialities such as ophthalmology do not have obvious trends. Seasonal trends are important as they can skew the analysis — if you do not look at the whole year, is the increase you have detected a real increase, or is it due to a summer bulge? When looking at long term trends it is useful to compare years on the same graph, so that changes between months can be separated from the year to year changes. An example can be found in figure 65, where waiting lists for several years are compared. Note that the newest line is stable — compared to an upward slope for the same months of previous years.

FIGURE 65
The waiting list compared year on year

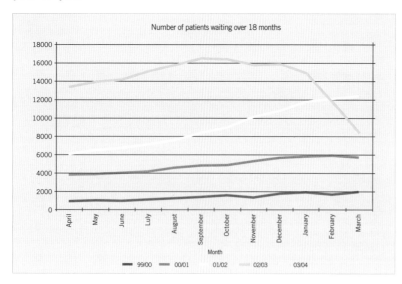

Conversion ratios

It is important to treat the elective process as an integrated whole. Increased activity at outpatient clinics may affect the flow on to the surgical waiting list, but simple conversion ratios may not give accurate predictions of future surgical demand.

With long waiting lists, an initiative clinic to remove patients from the tail of the waiting list where primary targeting lists have not previously been used, may deliver lower conversion ratios due to the nature of the patients who tend to accumulate at the end of waiting lists. Conversely, pre-screening of orthopaedic referrals by a physiotherapist may considerably reduce the number of new referrals onto the consultant outpatient waiting list. However, if the consultant continues to see the same number of outpatients, the ratio requiring surgery and thus the number flowing onto the inpatient waiting list, will increase substantially as those patients unlikely to proceed to surgery have been screened out.

Measuring follow-up demand

Many trusts and specialities have a problem with seeing outpatients at short notice. In response to the need to fit patients into full clinics two or less weeks into the future, Trusts have traditionally set aside appointment slots, or overbooked clinics at the last minute.

FIGURE 66
A typical ENT clinic — no slots available for the next seven weeks!

Understanding the workload.

Typically, Trusts understand demand for follow-up services even less than they understand demand for new referral slots. As a result, clinics are often overbooked and capacity is often exceeded by demand, leading to overcrowding and reduction in new referral capacity (figure 66). Even where information about the number of empty appointment slots is available when booking, one vital piece of information is missed out: how many more patients will be referred to that clinic between now and the clinic happening?

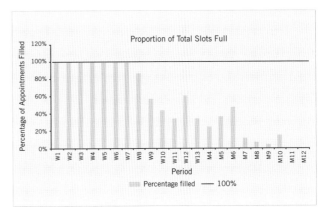

One way to understand what the demand will be on future services is to prospectively record every follow-up appointment made for a time period (preferably several months) and keep a track of how many one week, two week, three week etc. appointments are made each week. An alternative is to estimate the demand based on historical data. By analysing all the appointments made over an 18 month period, and calculating the time between the appointment and its predecessor, an estimate of appointment frequency can be made. The distribution for one ENT service, is shown in figure 67.

FIGURE 67
Number of weeks/months between a followup being made and the appointment

Note that 5% of appointments are made for one week, 5% for two weeks, 5% for three weeks etc. 25% of appointments are made for less than six weeks. In order to leave room for these patients, at six weeks the clinic should be only 75% full. The clinic in figure 66 is already full for the next seven weeks. Where will these patients be placed?

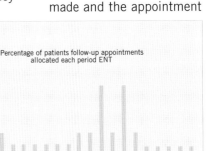

There needs to be a way to look at clinics and take account of the work that will come in, not only the work that has already come in. If that information is made available to clinicians, then they will be better able to make the decision about when to bring patients back — balancing clinical need with clinic availability. This can then be combined with a partial booking process for follow-up patients to reduce the last-minute overbooking and cancellation that is common today.

FIGURE 68A
Step 1

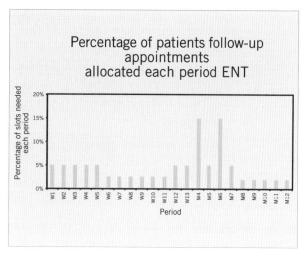

Percentage of patients follow-up appointments allocated each period ENT

Step 1: Plot the distribution...
Use as long a time frame as possible — the shorter the time you choose, the more under-represented the longer appointments will be, as either the first or the second appointment will be missing from the sample. Use a sample size of 18 months; more would be better!

Step 2: Convert to a cumulative graph...
The lower area represents the proportion of the clinic that should be filled, based on the distribution in the first graph. The upper area is the proportion needed to deal with the appointments 'yet to come'. The boundary between the upper and the lower is the proportion of the clinic that should be filled at any time. The boundary line represents 'full' if there is to be space available for any appointments yet to come.

FIGURE 68B
Step 2

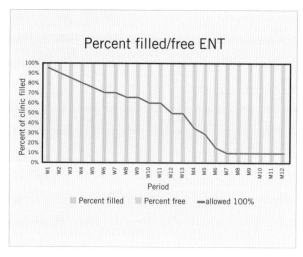

Percent filled/free ENT

Step 3: Plot your 'actuals'...
The jagged line represents the ENT clinic seen overleaf. As can be seen, there are times when it is above the boundary line — the clinic is over full. There are also times when the clinic is underfull for that week or month.

Step 4: Simplify the presentation...
The last graph 'flattens' the boundary line, setting it as '100%'. The jagged line becomes the series of vertical bars, showing over and underbooking against the new profile. This graph could be given to consultants or clinic staff to show where problems are predicted. Compare this graph for the clinic to figure 66.

Understanding demand for follow-up appointments will assist booking, and it will go a long way to improving the current chronic overbooking found in many clinics.

FIGURE 68C
Step 3

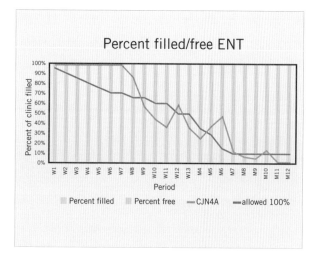

Percent filled/free ENT

FIGURE 68D
Step 4

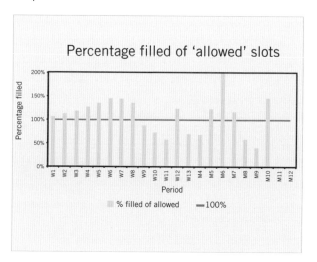

Percentage filled of 'allowed' slots

One of the main pressures on outpatient clinics is the volume of follow-up appointments. Regular follow-ups are seen as a high priority by many staff, often taking priority over new referrals into a clinic. It is common for new referrals to be cancelled when space for follow-ups is tight and this leads to increased waiting times for new referrals. Reducing follow-up attendances is the quickest way of increasing capacity within an outpatient clinic.

There are many ways to reduce follow-up attendance. In some cases, it is simply a matter of understanding the impact of follow-up appointments, and deciding as a multi-disciplinary team that the situation needs to be reviewed. In other cases, more formal approaches to reviewing the situation will be useful.

Understanding clinic profiles

It can be difficult to see the wood for the trees. Sometimes it is necessary to step back and review what is happening in outpatient clinics as a concerted exercise, rather than relying on perception and anecdotal evidence.

One way of doing this is to create a 'Week in the life of a clinic' to determine just what happens during a typical week.

The basic technique is to set up a data collection tool that can be applied to every patient seen in a department in a typical week. The data can be collected from the PAS, from patient records, and from checklists completed by staff during the clinic. Each of these will give a part of the picture:

CARDIFF AND VALE NHS TRUST

Nurse Practitioner in ENT

In common with many other Trusts in Wales, Cardiff and Vale has long waiting times for ENT and Audiological Medicine. The longest waiting patients are those with routine conditions whose needs inevitably have to be prioritised against those with urgent conditions including actual or suspected cancers.

A nurse practitioner was appointed in July 2002 with the specific objective of improving access times to the service. Following a period of training and development of care pathways and treatment protocols, she now works autonomously and provides assessment, diagnosis and treatment for patients referred from consultants and junior medical staff and GPs, and those she is able to select directly from the waiting list. Conditions the nurse practitioner is able to diagnose and treat include assessment of hearing loss, mastoid cavity care, aural care and treatment of infections, assessment for tonsillectomy and recurrent epistaxis.

The nurse practitioner's annual capacity is 2550 new outpatients, and 1000 follow-ups. For the patients she is able to treat, this has enabled a reduction in waiting times from 38 months to two months for one consultant, and to between 11 and three months for the other four.

Patient demographics including age/sex profiles, postcode analysis, referrer analysis.

Diagnosis and co-morbidities, number of times the patient has attended in the last year.

Who saw the patient, action taken, tests ordered, when the next appointment will be.

The information collected from these sources over a typical week should give enough data to be significant. Combining the data into a single database will allow collation across the different sources. The aim of the collation exercise should be to provide a picture of a typical cross section of patients seen in the department, and should help in answering a number of questions such as: what proportion of patients are local? What is the level of co-morbidity? What disease groups make up the highest proportion of frequent attenders? How many of the follow-up appointments were seen by junior staff, and what were the decisions taken?

The analysis may not provide any quick answers, but it will contribute to any subsequent improvement process. Without knowing the nature of the thing that is to be improved, there is a danger of concentrating on what seems obvious, or what 'everyone knows is the problem'. Having good data on the current situation is the first step to improvement.

This exercise can take a significant resource. Collection will involve looking at patient notes, and staff completing checklists for every patient they see during the week. The benefits are well worth the effort, as no-one can say that they are managing a service if they do not understand what is happening within that service.

Frequent attender analysis
A combination of analysis and action, this technique is a way of focussing efforts on the patients where the most return is likely.

From at least a year's data download from the PAS, do a frequency analysis of attendances by patient. The only data required for this is the patient number and the date of the outpatient appointment. Within a spreadsheet, a pivot table can be used to count the number of attendances by each patient. The pivot table can then be used to count the number of patients who had one appointment, two appointments and so on.

This is likely to show that the number of patients with significant multiple appointments is low, but that the number of appointments taken up by those patients is significant. In figure 69, which represents data for two years, one patient had 28 appointments, and three had 24 or 25 (one every month). In all, 18 patients (0.20%) accounted for 343 appointments (1.81%), below line 'A' while 125 patients (1.40%) had 10 or more appointments over the two years, representing 1,615 appointments (8.53%) below line 'B'.

FIGURE 69
Frequent attendance
data, 2 years clinics

Frequency of Attendance, 2 years data

Attendances	Number of patients	% of patients	Cumulative % of patients	Number of attendances	% of attendances	Cumulative % of attendances	
1	4761	53%	53%	4761	25%	25%	
2	2005	22%	76%	4010	21%	46%	
3	959	11%	86%	2877	15%	62%	
4	530	6%	92%	2120	11%	73%	
5	259	3%	95%	1295	7%	80%	
6	117	1%	96%	702	4%	83%	
7	92	1%	97%	644	3%	87%	
8	59	1%	98%	472	2%	89%	
9	48	1%	99%	432	2%	91%	
10	26	0%	99%	260	1%	93%	'B'
11	27	0%	99%	297	2%	94%	
12	19	0%	99%	228	1%	96%	
13	14	0%	100%	182	1%	97%	
14	10	0%	100%	140	1%	97%	
15	11	0%	100%	165	1%	98%	'A'
16	4	0%	100%	64	0%	99%	
16	6	0%	100%	102	1%	99%	
18	1	0%	100%	18	0%	99%	
19	3	0%	100%	57	0%	99%	
20	0	0%	100%	0	0%	99%	
21	0	0%	100%	0	0%	99%	
22	0	0%	100%	0	0%	99%	
23	0	0%	100%	0	0%	99%	
24	1	0%	100%	24	0%	100%	
25	2	0%	100%	50	0%	100%	
26	0	0%	100%	0	0%	100%	
27	0	0%	100%	0	0%	100%	
28	1	0%	100%	28	0%	100%	
29	0	0%	100%	0	0%	100%	
30	0	0%	100%	0	0%	100%	
	8955			18928			

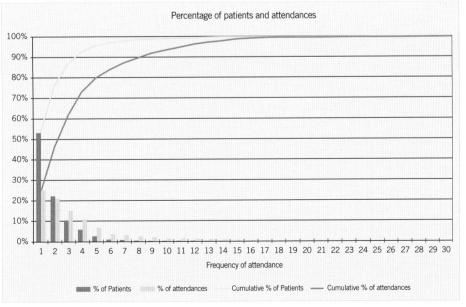

FIGURE 70
Distribution of patients and
appointments by frequency

6.4 Reducing follow-up demand   137

What can be done with this data? Pulling the patient records of the 18 patients and doing a clinical review may reveal changes to the care which would result in fewer appointments. Are these patients being best managed in outpatients? Would there be benefit in meeting with the patient's GP? By focussing on patients who are frequent attenders it may be possible to customise their care and improve the outcome, while also reducing the demand on outpatients. The key is identifying the small number of patients who are consuming relatively large amounts of clinic time, and then seeing if they can be managed better.

Use of 'SOS' appointments

Many departments now use self referral for follow-up rather than fixed appointments. This can be very effective in reducing both follow-up appointments and DNA rates in some situations. So called 'SOS' appointments can be used to advantage where the patient has a recurrent problem, where a procedure is being followed up, or where monitoring of a chronic condition can be undertaken in part by the patient.

Recurrent problems

This is the most common use of SOS appointments now. There is little point in regular follow-up of a condition which flares up from time to time, rather it is preferable to have rapid access to an appointment when the problem recurs.

Procedure follow-up

In many situations it is common to recall patients while they are recovering from a procedure. Often appointments are made on a regular basis, until the patient reports no further problems. This will always result in one more appointment than necessary (when the patient attends to report no symptoms) and often more than one appointment.

Informing the patient about the progression of recovery (through a patient pathway), and allowing the patient to make an appointment quickly if there is a deviation from the pathway or if the patient has any concerns, will mean that patients on the normal recovery path will not take up clinic time, which can then be devoted to those patients with problems.

Chronic condition monitoring

Patients with chronic conditions can also use SOS appointments, with the possibility of less frequent scheduled review.

In the case of chronic conditions, as with procedure follow-up, it is essential that the patient understands what events should trigger an appointment. Laminated cards with the events that should lead to an SOS appointment and instructions on how to make one are used with many patients.

Care must be taken with chronic conditions that have trigger events not apparent to the patient. Examples of these may be glaucoma or diabetic retinopathy in ophthalmology, or cholesterol levels in cardiology. In these cases, where the patient cannot monitor their own health, non-consultant monitoring can be used to reduce attendances in the outpatient clinic.

Follow-up referral protocols

Many attempts have been made to reduce referrals through the use of primary care referral protocols. Yet few departments have explicit protocols relating to the generation of a follow-up appointment although unnecessary follow-up appointments make up a higher proportion of clinic time than unnecessary new referrals.

Where junior staff review patients, the development and use of explicit protocols on the need to bring patients back to clinic will significantly reduce follow-up appointments. Junior staff have a tendency to bring patients back if in doubt — protocols make explicit when a patient should be brought back (or given an SOS appointment.

All departments should develop follow-up protocols for their major patient groups, and monitor their use.

'Carve out' is an insidious process that steals capacity before our eyes, while appearing to protect the capacity for those patients who need it. In complex processes like health, some carve out is inevitable, but it must be eliminated where it can be, and managed where it cannot.

What is carve out?

Carve out is a term given to circumstances where reserving some of a resource for one group reduces the resource available to another group. Carve out is seen every day. It is present in supermarket car parks (parent with child parking), in the supermarket itself (basket only queues), on the road (bus lanes) and in health. Health is the natural home of carve out — the NHS has adopted it as a solution to a problem, and in doing so created an even bigger problem.

How many queues are there?

In a typical outpatient clinic there are probably hundreds of queues. There are slots for new patients, there are slots for urgent new patients. There are postoperation slots and there are soon review slots. In some clinics the number of slots can run well into two digits. These slots are created in an attempt to balance out the capacity to match the patients coming through the clinic, but it is an endeavour doomed from the start. There is a very simple reason.

That many queues cannot be managed.

The odds that every week (or any week for that matter) the exact proportion of patients will match the available slots are minute. What happens instead is that there are empty slots, then the clinic is overbooked to fit the extra patients in. The schedule goes out of the window, and the flow of work is totally disrupted.

Banks worked this out some time ago: they have a single queue, feeding into multiple windows. The days when you joined one of multiple queues at the Post Office and cursed because the others were always moving faster are long gone.

What is the impact of carve-out?

Carve out wastes capacity. Figure 71 represents an outpatient clinic with a high degree of carve out — separate slots for each patient type, different clinics for different conditions. The lower, red line shows what the

FIGURE 71
With and without
carve out

Rheumatology comparison between Generic and Specialist Clinics
Capacity vs Demand

Capacity — Demand — Capacity backlog with generic booking — Capacity backlog with carveout booking

waiting list would have been if each patient was booked into the next available slot instead of the allocated speciality slot.

Dealing with carve out

Some carve out is necessary and has benefits in spite of the negative impact on waiting times. Two such examples are carve out to reserve space for urgent patients in partial booking, and carve out to allow clinical subspecialisation. The important thing is to allow the benefits and manage the carve out to minimise its effects.

Dealing with the 10 day waits

Partial booking allocates patients to clinics about four weeks before the appointment. There is a need to reserve some capacity for those patients that the Trust does not know about four weeks from the clinic.

As described on page 67 there are ways of managing this carve out so that it does not affect the waiting times for non-10 day patients. The key to resolving carve out in this case is to manage the impact of carve out.

Managing subspecialisation

The chapter on pooling in waiting lists gives methods that allow Trusts to deal with carve out caused by subspecialisation. Subspecialisation has benefits in improving skill mix in specialist areas. The carve out caused by subspecialisation must be managed, rather than trying to prevent it.

FIGURE 72
From a prioritised list to generic slots

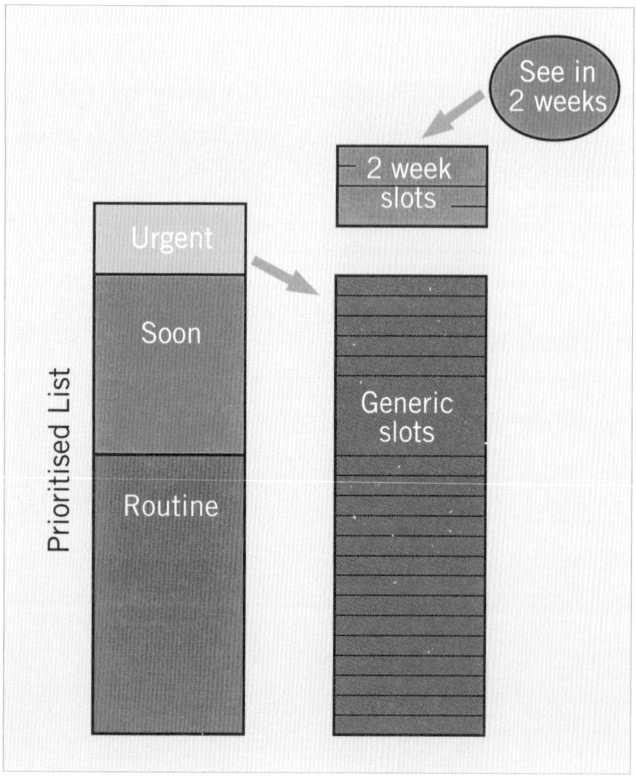

Prioritisation and carve out

It is important to distinguish between clinical prioritisation and carve out. While there are issues with the type of prioritisation used, if waiting lists are longer than a few weeks, some degree of prioritisation will be essential. The degree of prioritisation should be minimised, so that as few categories are used as are required to meet the need to see patients within clinical priority.

Accepting clinical prioritisation does not mean allocating carved out slots to each category of prioritisation. This is the key to managing carve out caused by prioritisation; prioritise a single list of patients, and then allocate those patients from the top of the list into non-differentiated slots in the clinic. 'Urgent' patients do not go into 'urgent' slots; 'soon' patients do not go into 'soon' slots and 'routine' patients are not booked into 'routine' slots. Instead all 'urgent', 'soon' and 'routine' patients are booked into generic outpatient slots.

No system works so well that you can assume it will work from day one, and continue to work. Ongoing monitoring and feedback to staff is as essential to the success of the improvement process as work going into the initial setup. There are a number of factors that must be carefully watched if the long term success of booking is to be maintained. These are Key Performance Indicators (KPIs).

Outpatient KPIs

Could not attend (CNA) delays

It is useful as a performance measure to be able to see what notice you are getting of CNAs. If CNAs are dated in the PAS, it is possible to report on the proportion of cancellations that are on the day of appointment or surgery (these appointments cannot be reused by another patient) as compared to those made early enough that the appointment time can be reused. This also allows you to compare the number of appointments or theatre minutes lost which were as a result of patient cancellations more than 24 hours in advance (pointing you to work on improving the short notice booking mechanisms in the appointment centre).

DNA Rates and cancellation rates

Regular (at least monthly) reporting on DNA rates and both patient and hospital cancellation rates is a must. This is the information required to convince staff that any new system works. It is important to flag those patients booked through the old system, and compare the rates to those managed through the new, in order to highlight the differences in those clinics where not every patient is booked.

How far ahead are we booking?

The time to the currently allocated phone date is vital information about potential workload. If your PAS calculates this information as is the case in our pilot, weekly reports by clinic enable you to see where wait times are getting longer or shorter, a simple and effective measure to assist in calculating capacity issues.

Are patients booked in 4 weeks?

Some Trust outpatient systems may not be able to implement the method for booking follow-up patients recommended in Chapter 3.3. If your system cannot be adapted, you will need to introduce KPIs to allow the monitoring of follow-up booking.

If the system sends 'phone now' letters 4 weeks prior to the original estimated appointment, weekly monitoring of the available slots is vital. We suggest a 'traffic light' system where you record which appointment date a phone booking is made.

If the appointments made in response to phone calls are four weeks away, then the clinic is in 'Green' and the system is performing well. There are two 'Amber' states. 'Amber and increasing' at five weeks means that there are more patients phoning than there are appointment slots, and the system must be watched closely to determine if this is a statistical fluctuation or a longer term trend. If it is a trend, the number of slots for follow-up will need monitoring. If statistical, the situation will right itself. Statistical variation may be caused by a single cancelled clinic.

In the 'Amber and decreasing' state, once again careful monitoring is in order. The same questions arise as to whether the decrease is statistical, or due to too few patients for the clinic slots.

'Red' states are more serious. At 'Red two weeks', measures need to be taken to: a) ensure that clinics are booked fully; and b) determine whether this is a worsening problem. If you have been monitoring you will know this from the work done during 'Amber', but now action is needed, and a predetermined course (bringing patients forward etc) put in place.

'Red six weeks' is an issue of a different sort. Action is needed here because we can now no longer give patients certainty, and urgent action is needed to pull the booking back to under six weeks. Once again, an action plan should be in place to respond.

Are we cancelling patients?

An important measure is the number of patients getting their appointment on the date they originally negotiated. Usually reported as hospital cancellations, this measure gives surety that the patient is getting the service promised.

Smooth running of clinics

The promise to clinicians was that booking would improve their quality of life in the clinics. Hard evidence about over / under booking, over / under run clinics, late starts and finishes will all help keep control of this area.

Clinic profiles

Annual review of all clinic profiles, or review whenever clinic procedures change, is vital. A system needs to be in place that monitors when each profile was last updated and when it is due for review. It is too easy for this to slip over time.

Elective waiting lists

There are a number of tools which can be used to monitor elective waiting lists. The two most important are monitoring the trends in numbers and waiting times, and monitoring the way in which patients are removed from the list for booking.

The monitoring of waiting lists, both in terms of numbers waiting and the length of waits, is best done through the use of SPC charts (see page 105). SPC charts will allow the detection of trends, and distinguish between trends and random variation. SPC charts for both the number of patients on the list and the number of patients waiting over a pre-set amount of time (e.g. 12 months) are essential.

How are patients booked?

The biggest problem with managing waiting lists is ensuring that the patients are removed in strict date order according to pre-determined clinical priority. There are several approaches to this.

How long did patients wait?

Report on the length of time each patient waited, and look at the distribution of waits. If patients are being booked in turn, all patients of the same clinical priority will have similar waits.

How long are patients waiting?

What is the shape of the waiting list? If patients are being taken in turn, it should have a level period followed by a steep drop, rather than a steady drop over time.

PTLS

The use of the Primary Target Rate and the Primary Targeting List Score as a way of monitoring treatment in chronological order is now standard across Wales, both within Trusts and as a national KPI. The tool is a simple and effective way of ensuring patients are treated in turn in any waiting list, and should be measured and reported for all elective services.

CPaT

The Modernisation Agency has put together a set of tools for monitoring waiting lists. See Chapter 2.5

Effective Use of Theatres

The Audit Commission in Wales Acute Hospital Portfolio[1] report states that in Wales:

- Patients wait longer than those in England to be admitted for routine surgical treatment;

- There is strong evidence that when more beds are available, more patients are placed on the waiting list;

- 10% patients have had their admission cancelled within a week of a planned operation;

- Only 70% of patients received their operation within a month of the original cancellation;

- There is variation in pre-assessment practices;

- Published waiting time data do not always reflect the full patient experience.

1 Acute Hospital Portfolio, No2. Audit Commission in Wales, 2001

It is recognised that Operating Theatre time is one of the most expensive resources that a trust has to manage and it is an extremely complicated task to ensure that all the correct equipment, stores and staff are assembled in the same place at the same time that the patient needs them.

The publication of the Modernisation Agency's Step Guide to Improving Operating Performance[1] was the culmination of an extensive project involving nine pilot sites in England. The project examined all aspects of Operating Theatre provision and the tools developed, along with the Step Guide itself, offers straightforward, step by step advice to improving theatre services. Innovations in Care were involved in the revising of the final draft of the document and there was a recognition that the issues identified were common to Wales and that the solutions suggested would be as valid. It was agreed to adopt the document as the main reference document for the Innovations in Care All Wales Theatre Programme.

The Step Guide

Step 1: Planning & management

Trusts are encouraged to set up properly agreed management structures that have sufficient authority to make the decisions necessary to ensure optimum use of theatre capacity. Timely and accurate information is key to informing the decisions that must be made to ensure optimum performance. This is reinforced in the Audit Commission Acute Hospital Portfolio report on Operating Theatres[2] that identified that information is key to effective management of theatres. As in the Step Guide, the NLIAH recommends planning and management structures to support effective planning and management of operating theatre performance, including implementation of systems to report regularly on key performance indicators.

The first chapter of the guide also covers:

■ Actions for NHS Trust Boards.

■ The role and membership of the Theatre Management Group.

■ Theatre policy documents.

■ Examples of effective practice.

One of the key recommendations is that the importance of theatre management is underlined by nominating an Executive Director to be responsible for theatre performance.

Step 2: Diagnosis & analysis

The Theatre programme in Wales has developed its own Key Performance Indicators that reflect the areas that management should have knowledge of on a regular (monthly) basis. These indicators build on the information already submitted by trusts in the Cancelled Operation data. Analysis of both will identify key areas for trusts to focus their efforts on to ensure improvement to the service. An example of the type of outcome chart is shown in figure 73.

1 *Step Guide for Improving Operating Theatre Performance (including pre-operative assessment for inpatients and day surgery).* Modernisation Agency, 2002

2 *Acute Hospital Portfolio, Report on Operating Theatres.* Audit Commission in Wales, 2003

The sharing of this information between Trusts has allowed benchmarking and identification of areas of good practice and it is recommended that trusts continue to meet with each other on a regular basis to ensure the continuation of this 'shared learning'.

FIGURE 73
Utilisation of operating hours

The Step Guide also contains diagnostic tools that examine the patient experience and staff satisfaction. The NLIAH recommends that Trusts undertake these surveys and discuss the results with colleagues across Wales and in England.

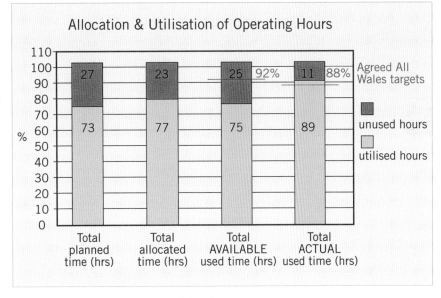

Step 3: Improving operating theatre performance

Where areas of concern are identified the NLIAH will provide training in process mapping techniques to enable staff to highlight the bottlenecks and constraints in a system and be able to redesign the service using Plan Do Study Act cycles to ensure measurable improvement.

The Modernisation Agency Step Guide divides this chapter into three key areas:

1. Patient experience;

2. Human Resources;

3. Elective & Emergency surgery.

It must be recognised when attempting to improve Operating Theatre services that some of the key impacts are often outside the department. So it is vital that all stakeholders in the Operating Theatre services are identified and involved in any improvement strategy. As with the other sections of this guide it is recommended that a whole system approach is taken when making improvement.

Step 4: Scheduling

The main areas that affect effective use of theatre time are scheduling and internal arrangements for getting the patient to the right theatre at the right time. Effective pre-operative assessment has a double effect on theatre efficiency by ensuring that cancellations are minimised and therefore ensuring that utilisation is increased.

Overbooking of theatre sessions will have a detrimental effect on cancellation rates. It is the second most important cause of cancellations due to non-clinical reasons: in the first quarter of 2003, over 370 operations were cancelled due to list over-runs. This is where effective and timely scheduling is key. Surgeons and theatre management teams must make use of available information to ensure theatre sessions are accurately planned. Prospective lists should be published with adequate time or early notification must be given of special needs to ensure theatres have the correct equipment available.

GOOD PRACTICE POINT

Improving Theatre Utilisation

All Trust should complete the Self Assessment Checklist that is included in the Step Guide for Improving Theatre Performance.
This will provide a baseline assessment against the standard and will highlight areas of compliance and non compliance from which trusts can target their improvement action plans.

Dermatology Nurse Specialists

As a result of the long waiting times in Dermatology, Dermatology nurses within Conwy & Denbighshire NHS Trust have developed their roles to relieve some of the demands on the service.

A nurse-led acne clinic has been developed, seeing patients directly from the waiting list, which has reduced the waiting times from 18 months to 6 months within a 6-month period.

Those patients prescribed Roaccutane require close monitoring and support. A nurse-led monitoring clinic has been established which fulfils this need, allowing more time for doctors to see patients from waiting lists.

SOS patients are given an access phone number for short-notice appointments.

Teledermatology

To improve access to the service, a Dermatology nurse was appointed in September 2002, with the focus of introducing teledermatology to the Trust. Following an introductory period of training, planning and developing protocols, teledermatology clinics have been introduced to three peripheral sites on a 'store and forward' basis. Images are viewed by a consultant Dermatologist, and the suspected skin cancer referrals prioritised accordingly. Initially, this has been used as a triage imaging assessment tool of skin lesions, and not a substitute for consultation.

As a result, a nurse-led lesion-screening clinic has been developed, allowing greater access to the specialty for routine conditions, thus reducing waiting times by a quarter over the last few months from 24 to less than 18 months, with a target waiting time of 12 months by March 2004.

Systems of work must be examined to ensure that delays in patient transfers are minimised.

Electronic copies of the following documents are also available on www.modernnhs.nhs.uk/theatreprogramme

- Step Guide to Improving Operating Performance[1]

- Theatre programme diagnostic tools & user manuals[2]

[1] *Step Guide for Improving Operating Theatre Performance (including preoperative assessment for inpatients and day surgery)* http://www.portal.modern.nhs.uk/sites/crosscutting/access/Access%20Document%20Library/1/Theatres/Step%20Guide/Complete%20Step%20Guide.pdf

[2] *Step Guide for Improving Operating Theatre Performance (including preoperative assessment for inpatients and day surgery)* www.portal.modern.nhs.uk/sites/crosscutting/access/Access%20Document%20Library/1/Theatres/Step%20Guide/Complete%20Step%20Guide.pdf

Conclusions

The purpose of key performance indicators is to ensure that everything is running smoothly. It is far easier to keep on top of the problems than to fix them later.

Do not be afraid of setting up too many monitoring tools. It is easier to set up tools to monitor more than you think will be necessary and then to stop the ones that are less use than to have to set up new measures six months down the track because the process has gone wrong. Overmeasure at first, and pare down the tools over time.

Avoid using KPIs as a way of imposing performance targets. While KPIs can be (and are) used this way, the real value of KPIs is in allowing the staff in a service to look at their performance and see what is really happening.

Statistical Process Control

Statistical Process Control (SPC) can help in virtually all aspects of managing healthcare. From monitoring of waiting times for a Trust to monitoring prescribing on a ward, SPC provides a way of separating the 'information' from the 'noise' so that managers and clinicians can understand what is going on. Too often decisions are made without knowing whether changes in data are due to actions taken, or merely due to chance.

The time has come to reclaim the benefits of this methodology and use the tools to understand and monitor the work we do on a daily basis. To help in this, this chapter abandons the nomenclature traditionally used in statistical process control methodology. To assist those who are familiar with the older jargon, there is a short glossary on the next page.

Ignoring time: The curse of the monthly report

Most healthcare organisations manage through monthly reporting. These reports present data for the past month (often several weeks after the end of the time period) and probably a year to date position, including a target.

Unfortunately, a monthly progress report shows little about the future. Indeed, managing by the monthly report has been likened to driving a car by watching the road in the rear view mirror. To manage future events, you must predict the future. The best approach to prediction is analysis of past trends.

The best way to display trends in data is the run chart — plotting weekly or monthly values as a time sequence. Run charts are a significant improvement over traditional reporting techniques, because they introduce the concept of changes over time.

Unfortunately, in order to manage a trend, it is necessary to go one step further. Is the change in the run chart due to a change in the process, or is it simply due to random fluctuation? To do this, the trend must be separated from the noise resulting from random variation. Much damage can be done by assuming a monthly change is the break in a trend, or represents a change resulting from action taken last month, when in fact it represents the effect of routine variation caused by random factors. This is where process behaviour charts come in.

The process behaviour chart

Process behaviour charts are a type of run chart. The aim of a run chart is to look for changes in performance over time. The aim of a process behaviour chart is to show whether the changes seen in the run chart are as a result of routine variation in the process, or the result of exceptional variation, indications that something in the process has changed. From the separation of routine and exceptional variation it is possible to determine whether the changes in data represent changes in performance or simply the normal variability of the system.

Figure 74 illustrates this problem. It is a run chart showing the time sequence from April 2000 to March 2001, and the number of patients waiting over 18 months for an outpatient appointment. The graph shows a drop in March, which is against the trend for the previous year. Does this drop represent a real change, a one off event, or random variation?

It is difficult to see changes in the trends in figure 74. They can be made clearer by plotting the **change** from month to month, rather than the actual values. This has been done in figure 75. A constant trend will now be shown as a horizontal line, and the difficulty of estimating changes in slope are removed.

We have adopted most of the recommendations of Donald J Wheeler in this section[1]

Instead of control chart we use process behaviour chart.

Instead of in control process we use predictable process.

Instead of out of control process we use unpredictable process.

Instead of an in control point we use a point inside the limits.

Instead of an out of control point we use a point outside the limits.

Instead of control limits we use natural process limits.

Instead of common cause variation we use routine variation.

Instead of special cause variation we use exceptional variation.

We have chosen to remain with Statistical Process Control (SPC) rather than Wheeler's Methods of Continual Improvement because we feel the term too encompassing of other tools used in quality improvement.

Figure 75 shows that the change in numbers waiting from month to month does vary between -200 and +450, and it also shows that March 2001 represents the first point at which there is a negative value — a reduction in the waiting list. Is this reduction real, or simply random fluctuation? The answer can be provided by converting the run chart to a process behaviour chart.

Creating the process behaviour chart

To convert this run chart to a process behaviour chart, some calculations are necessary, and some information must be added.

1. Calculate the average change. Exclude the March 2001 data from the averaging process as the purpose is to see if this is outside the normal range. The average line (shown on figure 76 as the dotted line) is therefore the average of the values from May 2000 to February 2001.

2. Calculate the average moving range (AMR). The moving range is the difference between each value and the next. If the difference is a negative number, ignore the sign. In this example the AMR is 150.

3. Multiply the AMR by 2.66 (150 X 2.66 = 400). 2.66 is a constant, derived for this purpose.

4. The upper natural process limit is the value from step 3 added to the average (206 + 400 = 606).

5. The lower natural process limit is the value from step 3 subtracted from the average (206 - 400 = -194).

1 *Understanding Variation: The Key to Managing Chaos.* Wheeler, Donald J, 1993

These limits can now be plotted on figure 76. They are represented as the red lines.

The natural process limits represent the range within which the process can expected to vary. Any variation outside these limits will indicate that the process has in some way changed.

Interpretation of the process behaviour chart

The natural process limits represent the range within which variation is routine. If a point falls outside those limits, it is due to exceptional causes — either to some one-off exceptional event, or a change in the process in some way. When the data fall outside the range shown on the charts, you will know that something has been done that has affected the number of long waiting patients.

The March 2001 value, while low and the first reduction seen, does not fall outside the natural process limits. While the reduction may be due to extra end of year work, there is no reason to put the reduction down to anything other than routine variation within the process.

FIGURE 74
The run chart of the numbers waiting

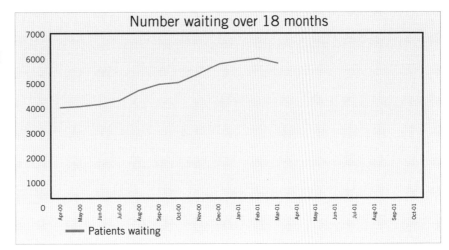

FIGURE 75
The run chart of change from month to month

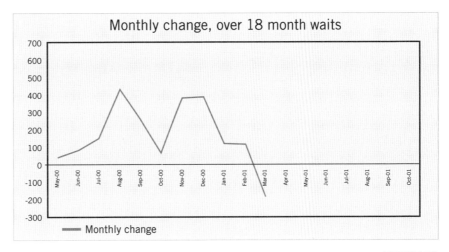

FIGURE 76
The process behaviour chart of change month to month

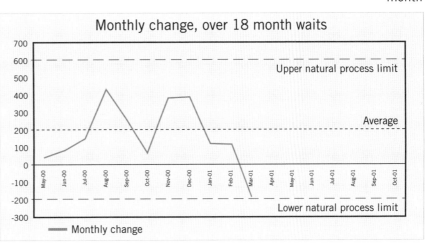

FIGURE 77
The process behaviour
chart extended to October
2001

Extending the series

What happens if we extend the graph? On Figure 77, data through to October 2001 have been added.

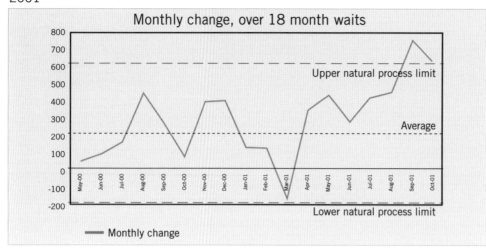

Both September and October 2001 are outside the natural process limits on figure 77. This indicates that these two months represent a change in the process. Something has led to an increase in the rate at which the number of over 18 month waits is growing. But when did the increased trend start? Was it in September, or was it earlier and took until September to exceed the limits?

There are three tests of a change in behaviour in a process behaviour chart. Each of these tests indicates that something outside the normal course of variation has occurred.

FIGURE 78
The run chart extended to
2001

1. The appearance of a point outside the natural process limits has already been covered. A single point (rather than a series of points) outside the range could represent a one-off exceptional variation, due to either a change in the process or an outside cause that affected only that month. A single point should therefore be regarded with caution as an indication that the process has been changed.

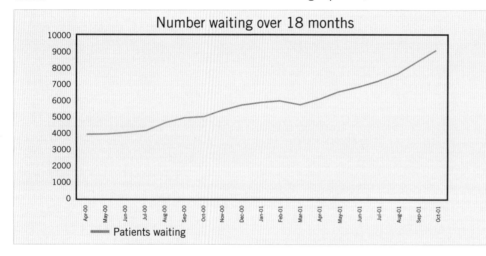

2. A run of eight or more points on one side of the average line. In figure 77, all the points from April 2001 are on the upper side of the average, and if the November data were also above 206 this would satisfy the test that a change existed from April 2001. At present it does not. This test will pick up relatively small changes in the trend, but it needs a long period (8 time intervals) to show up.

3. Three of four consecutive points are closer to one of the natural process limits than the average. On figure 77, May 01, July 01 and August 01 are all closer to the upper natural process limit than the average. This test has been met, and indicates a change in the process from earlier than September 01 when the first point is outside the upper natural process limit. It indicates that there has been a change in the process in place since around May 2001.

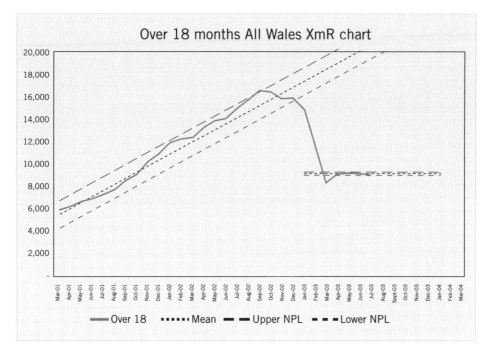

FIGURE 79
A more complex
behaviour chart, showing
different stages in a
process, with the upper
limits recalculated after a
major change in the
process behaviour. This
chart also shows a sloping
set of process limit lines

Figure 78 extends figure 74 over the same date range, and shows that the slope on the chart from March 2001 is steeper than prior to that date. This supports the proposition that something has changed across Wales since April 2001, but the process behaviour charts confirm the significance of the change.

It would be possible to generate the process behaviour chart on the raw data in figure 74. To do this, as there is a trend upwards in the data, the average line needs to incorporate the steady state increase. This can be done by creating an 'average' line that is a 'best fit' and calculating the natural process limits either side of the best fit line. Although this is possible (see March 01 to September 02 in figure 79) it is more complicated.

Use of process behaviour charts

Process behaviour charts are used to separate the 'noise' from the 'information' in a data series. They can be used to analyse trends and make reliable predictions about the future. They can also be used to monitor performance and determine whether performance changes are real or simply an artifact of the variation in the system.

More importantly, process behaviour charts can be used to analyse and monitor changes made as part of an improvement process. As part of the PDSA cycle (change through experimentation) process behaviour charts can be set up to monitor the processes that are being changed. It will then be possible to determine whether a change to the process (as part of a Plan Do Study Act cycle) has in fact led to a change in the performance of the process. Without using process behaviour charts to monitor performance of the Plan Do Study Act cycle it will not be possible to determine accurately whether the outcome is a result of the change, or simply the effect of variation.

Wheeler's principles for understanding data

First principle:
No data have meaning apart from their context

Second principle:
While every data set contains noise, some data sets contain signals. Therefore, before you can detect a signal within a data set, you must first filter out the noise.

One stop clinics: Office gynaecology

As a result of the long inpatient and outpatient waiting times in Gynaecology, the Obstetric and Gynaecology Directorate within the Conwy and Denbighshire NHS Trust have expanded the One Stop Clinic to reduce the waiting list times. The main aims of the One Stop Clinic are as follows :

- *Investigation and management of postmenopausal bleeding*
- *Investigation and management of menorrhagia*
- *Investigation of female urinary incontinence*

The clinic is run every Monday and every other Thursday and led by a Consultant Obstetrician and Gynaecologist. This consultant currently runs a rapid access postmenopausal bleeding clinic, other 'see and treat' procedures carried out within the One Stop Clinic are :

- *Hysteroscopies*
- *Biopsies*
- *Scans*
- *Insertion of Mirena coils*

With the successful introduction of the One Stop Clinic waiting lists have been reduced dramatically over the past twelve months, thus reducing pressure on the service. Future aims are to double the capacity for combined colposcopy and hysteroscopy procedures.

Critical Chain: managing projects effectively

This chapter covers the principles of the critical chain approach to project management. Critical chain is a project management application of the **Theory of Constraints**, developed by Eliyahu Goldratt and first introduced in *The Goal*[1]. A good first introduction to critical chain project management can be found in *Critical Chain*[2] by Goldratt.

Why are projects so difficult?
There is nothing so sure than the truth that projects will fail. In the development of software, the building industry, health, education, in all walks of life, in all countries, projects fail.

Of 80 major projects started in the US Department of Energy between 1980 and 1996, 31 terminated before they were completed, after $10billion had been spent. Only 15 of the 80 were completed (and three of those do not do what they were intended) while the remaining 34 were ongoing[3].

The phenomenon of the failing project is so well understood and so widely acknowledged that a quick search of the internet will turn up thousands of examples of the 'Laws of Project Management' (one version can be found on page 156). Despite this widespread acceptance of failure, we continue to plan projects, execute projects and excuse failed projects on a daily basis. Projects are a fact of life in the NHS as in most other workplaces, and what we really need is an approach that improves the likelihood that we will succeed.

Over the years methodologies have been developed to improve success. Tools like PRINCE2 have been developed to break projects down into smaller steps, to increase and improve reporting, to standardise documentation and to aid in clarifying scope. Despite all these tools, all the PRINCE2 training, and all the additional effort placed on monitoring, delivery of the full scope of projects on time and within budget continues to be an elusive, rarely seen, goal.

The three key parameters of a project
When we undertake a project we expend resources to achieve a goal within the boundary of three parameters (figure 80). These are scope, cost and schedule, and they are the key to successful project delivery.

1 *The Goal*, Goldratt and Cox, 2004

2 *Critical Chain*, Goldratt 1997

3 *Critical Chain Project Management*, Leach, 2000

LAW 1: *No major project is ever completed on time, within budget, with the same staff that started it, nor does the project do what it is supposed to do. It is highly unlikely that yours will be the first.*

> *Corollary 1: The benefits will be smaller than initially estimated, if estimates were made at all.*
>
> *Corollary 2: The system finally installed will be completed late and will not do what it is supposed to do.*
>
> *Corollary 3: It will cost more but will be technically successful.*

LAW 2: *One advantage of fuzzy project objectives is that they let you avoid embarrassment in estimating the corresponding costs.*

LAW 3: *The effort required to correct a project that is off course increases geometrically with time.*

> *Corollary 1: The longer you wait the harder it gets.*
>
> *Corollary 2: If you wait until the project is completed, it's too late.*
>
> *Corollary 3: Do it now regardless of the embarrassment.*

LAW 4: *The project purpose statement you wrote and understand will be seen differently by everyone else.*

> *Corollary 1: If you explain the purpose so clearly that no one could possibly misunderstand, someone will.*
>
> *Corollary 2: If you do something that you are sure will meet everyone's approval, someone will not like it.*

LAW 5: *Measurable benefits are real. Intangible benefits are not measurable, thus intangible benefits are not real.*

> *Corollary 1: Intangible benefits are real if you can prove that they are real.*

LAW 6: *Anyone who can work effectively on a project part-time certainly does not have enough to do now.*

> *Corollary 1: If a boss will not give a worker a full-time job, you shouldn't either.*
>
> *Corollary 2: If the project participant has a time conflict, the work given by the full-time boss will not suffer.*

LAW 7: *The greater the project's technical complexity, the less you need a technician to manage it.*

> *Corollary 1: Get the best manager you can. The manager will get the technicians.*
>
> *Corollary 2: The reverse of corollary 1 is almost never true.*

LAW 8: *A carelessly planned project will take three times longer to complete than expected. A carefully planned project will only take twice as long.*

> *Corollary 1: If nothing can possibly go wrong, it will anyway.*

LAW 9: *When the project is going well, something will go wrong.*

> *Corollary 1: When things cannot get any worse, they will.*
>
> *Corollary 2: When things appear to be going better, you have overlooked something.*

LAW 10: *Project teams detest weekly progress reporting because it so vividly manifests their lack of progress.*

LAW 11: *Projects progress rapidly until they are 90 percent complete. Then they remain 90 percent complete forever.*

LAW 12: *If project content is allowed to change freely, the rate of change will exceed the rate of progress.*

LAW 13: *If the user does not believe in the system, a parallel system will be developed. Neither system will work very well.*

LAW 14: *Benefits achieved are a function of the thoroughness of the post-audit check.*

> *Corollary 1: The prospect of an independent post-audit provides the project team with a powerful incentive to deliver a good system on schedule within budget.*

LAW 15: *No law is immutable.*

[1] http://ifaq.wap.org/science/lawprojman.html 2005

7.1 Critical Chain: Managing projects effectively

Scope

The scope of the project defines the minimum standard that must be achieved. Normally we think of scope from a planning perspective of 'what is in and what is out', but this is simply another way of saying that the scope is what we must deliver.

Clarity around the scope of the project is very important if we are to avoid 'project scope drift' where things are added to the project on an ad-hoc basis over time, and the final delivered result bears little if any resemblance to the original plan. Lack of clarity around scope also leads to project failure, as the scope is allowed to expand yet the resources available to deliver are not.

Scope is best thought of as *the minimum standard we have to deliver.*

Cost

Cost of projects is often ignored in the NHS, as many costs are hidden. We may not take account of staff time (other than the project manager), we may hide costs within other budgets, or we may use the project budget to cover other running costs. However projects should include, as part of the proposal and part of the evaluation, a cost/benefit analysis — and you cannot do a cost/benefit analysis without understanding the costs.

Cost for the project is *the maximum cost that must not be exceeded.*

Schedule

Schedule is the time available for a project. Time is a valuable commodity for any project, and it is the commodity that most easily runs out. In NHS improvement projects, where cost is less visible than other elements, it is the balance between scope and schedule that is most at risk.

The schedule represents the *maximum time we have to deliver the scope.* The majority of this chapter concentrates on how we manage time within our projects.

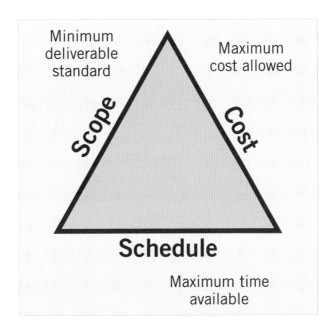

FIGURE 80
The project management pyramid

FIGURE 81
A PERT chart post-it

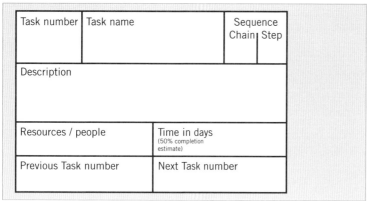

Task number	Task name		Sequence Chain⏐Step
Description			
Resources / people		Time in days (50% completion estimate)	
Previous Task number		Next Task number	

Planning the project: PERT, Gantt, and the critical path

An important part of any project plan is organising the steps. There are a number of tools available to do this, the most dangerous being Microsoft Project© which generates Gantt charts. As with many software programmes, the ability to generate precise Gantt charts looks impressive, but an ability to use Project© no more makes a person a project manager than an ability to use Microsoft Word© makes them an author.

There are three steps to producing a meaningful project plan. First, list the tasks. Second, estimate the time each will take. Third, put them into some order which makes the overall project schedule as short and realistic as possible. Once this is done, the project is planned. Then, and only then, if necessary type the tasks into Microsoft Project©.

The best way to plan the project is to sit with the team and list all the possible tasks, placing each on a 'post-it' note. Pre-printed note pads which contain a format for project planning are useful (figure 81). For each task listed in the project, complete the post-it, including the task, the resources needed, and the time estimate (we will come onto the issues associated with task times shortly.) Once the tasks are all listed on the post-its, they can be placed on a board in the order the tasks need to be completed. The relationships between the tasks are now clear, and the PERT Chart is completed (see figure 82).

FIGURE 82
A PERT Chart

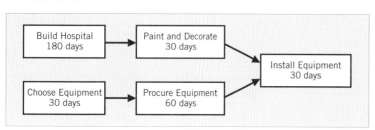

The Critical Path

Once the relationships are in place, and the sequence of all steps is worked out, it may become clear that there are multiple streams of events. It is rare for a project to consist of a single linear sequence of tasks. In every project however, there will be a critical path; the sequence of events that determines how long the overall project will take. In the example given on this page, there are two sequences of events, each consisting three boxes. The upper sequence takes a total of 240 days; the lower, 120 days. The upper sequence is therefore the critical path, as it determines the total length of the project. Delays on the lower path can be accommodated without affecting the overall project finish time.

FIGURE 83
A Critical Path

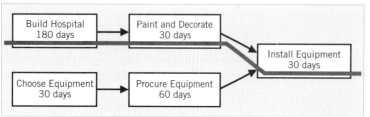

The Gantt Chart

The Gantt chart graphically adds the element of time to the PERT chart. Just as PERT charts are familiar to those who develop their project plans using post-its and whiteboards, Gantt charts are the preserve of the Microsoft Project© users. The primary difference between the PERT and Gantt chart is that in the Gantt chart, each box is sized according to the length of the task, and there is a horizontal time axis. The Gantt chart for the example project is shown in figure 84A. There is one problem with this chart however.
The concept of late start is illustrated here. Since the lower sequence of events takes 120 days less, the lower sequence can start 120 days into the project. This makes financial sense, as it would be 'poor planning' to have all the equipment ready three months before the building was ready. But what does the late start do to the critical path? Now both paths are critical — once the lower path starts at day 120, it too is critical to the project, and any delay on this path will now delay the project end date. As every event is now critical, project management and monitoring becomes even more complex, and there is much higher risk of failure.

An alternative is to place the delay as 'safety', by starting the lower path early (see figure 84B). This reduces the number of critical elements in the project.

It also increases cost (by requiring earlier payment for the equipment) and means that the equipment needs storing. The balancing of early start / late start is one of the many dilemmas in project management, and one of the reasons projects fail.

Where did all the time go?
Managing improvement programmes in the NHS is about managing time. Time is the most important resource we have available to us, and it is the one we are least able to manage successfully.

To understand the problems we have with managing time in projects, we must first understand the impact of variation and the concept of 'safety'

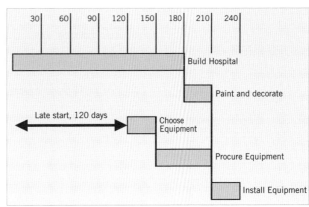

FIGURE 84A
A Gantt Chart
(with late start)

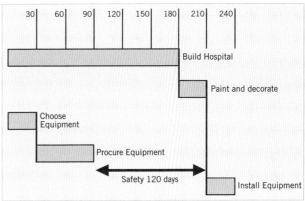

FIGURE 84B
A Gantt Chart
(with early start)

Variation

How long does it take to drive from Cardiff to Bangor? In a way, this is a nonsensical question because it has so many possible answers. If we ask in the context of how good our cars are then the estimates are likely to be low — people compete around how fast they can travel the distance. If we are estimating how long we need to leave to complete the journey, optimists will give a smaller estimate than pessimists. Everyone knows that there are any number of factors involved — weather, time of day, time of year. There are also the imponderables — road works, tractors, camper-vans. How much weight we give to these factors depends on our previous experiences. The longest estimate is likely to result if we make it clear that the reason for getting to Bangor on time is very important — a vital meeting, a job interview, a wedding. In these cases, we want to assign a high degree of certainty that we will arrive in time, and we will allow a lot of 'safety' time to allow for all the conceivable delays that may occur.

The probability of completing the journey within the predicted time can be represented graphically as a log normal distribution (figure 85). The area under the graph represents the probability that the completion time will fall within the time on the horizontal axis.

For example, Time 'A' represents 50% probability. For the particular journey, if we allow 'A' amount of time, there is a 50% chance that we will get there on time. To achieve greater certainty (eg 80% chance of getting there on time) we need to allow time 'B', and for even more assurance, a 90% chance of arriving on time for that very important meeting, we allow time 'C'.

The problem arises with the shape of the log normal curve. The long tail on the graph means that for a relatively small increase in certainty, say 10% (from 80% to 90%) we need to add a large amount of time. As a rough estimate, 80% certainty can be achieved by doubling the 50% estimate, 90% by tripling the 50% estimate.

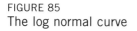
FIGURE 85
The log normal curve

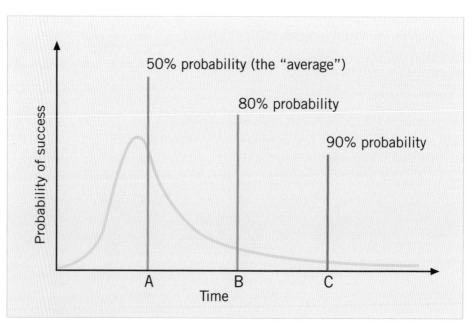

Projects must not fail! When calculating the time we will need to complete a task, it is unreasonable to set a time that means there is a 50% chance of failure. The more important the project, the more important the task, the more important it is to finish on time. Thus safety appears. Safety is the buffer between 50% completion and a higher degree of certainty that the project will be completed. And safety margins are huge. At 90% certainty, the safety can represent 2/3 of the available project time (figure 86).

The first thing to note when discussing safety is that people do not discuss safety! In general, project managers do not explicitly add double the likely time a task will take to the end of their estimate to ensure success — it is just part of the normal estimating process. Everyone puts it into their estimates, no-one admits to it, and no-one explicitly discusses it.

Where does the safety come from? In many projects the planned time is made almost entirely of safety. Each task estimate in the plan is likely to have safety estimates to the 90% level. Extra safety may be added to the overall project plan by the project manager once the individual task estimates are in. Every layer of management is likely to add additional safety to protect their reputation, and finally the project manager may add additional safety, knowing that someone higher up may cut back the time for the project because it is now too long.

So if there is so much safety in the project plan, why do projects continue to fail to meet deadlines? Where does that safety margin go? At 90%, almost every conceivable contingency must be covered — yet as has already been shown, projects continue to fail.

After so much safety has been added to the project that it now makes up by far the majority of the time the project will take, one of the ironies is that it is managed so badly. There are a several reasons for this.

Wasting safety: the curse of traditional project management
There are all sorts of ways to waste the safety that has been added to the project.

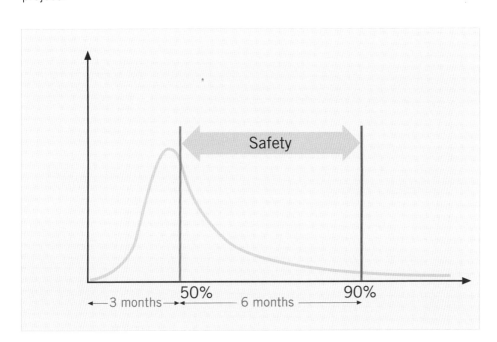

FIGURE 86
Safety

Milestones

Milestones represent significant points in a project. They are a useful way of identifying how far through the project is, as they will be clearly identified achievements. From this perspective, milestones are very useful.

For traditional project management, milestones have another, more significant value. Milestones are used to ensure that projects are completed on time. Dates are attached to milestones, and achievement of milestones by the target date is seen as the most important measure of progress. Projects which are critical are likely to have many intermediate milestones, so that those monitoring the project are able to assure that the project is 'on track'.

There is only one milestone where the date matters for a project: the final completion date. Dates for intermediate milestones are met by adding safety to every step along the way — in fact treating the achievement of milestones as projects in their own right. The more pressure to meet intermediate milestones, the larger the amount of safety that will be added at each step. What we are doing is trying to protect the project by protecting each step in the project!

This should give concern to those familiar with the Theory of Constraints approach to improvement. Adding safety to every step to ensure all milestones are met is the project equivalent of 'keeping all the machines running at full speed' — when what is needed is to identify the constraint in the system, and optimise that. What we do by creating milestones is ensure that safety is lost throughout the project, and it is never regained.

Delays accumulate; advances do not

When a step in the project over-runs, there is pressure from subsequent steps to extend deadlines. This is perfectly reasonable, after all if the time wasn't required for the subsequent step, it wouldn't have been allocated in the project plan. This means that where delays occur, they have the effect of delaying the whole project timeline. But what about the early finishes? If the estimates are all including safety to allow for a 90% probability of completion, there must be times (90% of the time) when the project step is finished before its target date.

What happens when a step finishes early? Perhaps the most obvious thing is that the people who are responsible for the next step will not be ready to start work. There is a project plan that shows them commencing their step in five days, and they have other work they are doing until then. Even if the work is handed over, they may not be able to just stop everything and start work early.

Secondly, if you finish early, what is the incentive to hand the work over? If you finish a report early, you are likely to set it aside to 'tidy up' some more between now and the deadline. An early completion just means that you have more time to tinker with the completed product.

Thirdly, reporting an early finish is one sure way of getting your time estimates cut in the future. If it is clear that you completed the work in $2/3$ of the available time, in the next project you are going to have less time to complete the work — after all there is pressure to reduce completion times, and where better to trim the schedule but in areas where it is known that they have taken less time in the past?

The Student Syndrome

There is another very human way of wasting safety and ensuring failure at a step. In *Critical Chain* Goldratt refers to this as the *student syndrome.*

The student syndrome (the term comes from the student approach to completing assignments, although it is pervasive in all work environments) is very simple:

- **We pad each step of the process so that we will have plenty of time.**
  We argue for 'realistic' deadlines and, for us, realistic means that we will have a 90% chance of completing the task (essay, report) in the time negotiated.

- **We know we have plenty of time, so we delay starting.** After all, we have allowed for plenty of safety, so there is no real pressure to start the task, and there are other higher priorities at the moment.

- **We start late and we run out of time.** Because all the safety was used up before we started, and because we are optimists and believe the task can be completed in the 50% time, when a problem arises (as by definition it will 50% of the time) there is now no safety to allow for the delay — and we miss the deadline!

Multitasking

Another way of wasting time is through multitasking. Once again this may appear to be counter-intuitive, but the impact on projects is easily seen. Multitasking is often seen as efficient; after all, if a person or resource works solely on one project at a time, there may be times when the resource is idle. Multitasking means that there is always some work that can be underway.

The problem of multitasking comes when one of the tasks is on the critical path of a project. If a person or department is providing some input into an external project (for example the Information Department may need to provide a report) and that step (providing the report) is on the critical path of a project, multitasking will inevitably lead to delays in the project. This is illustrated in figures 86A-86C.

FIGURE 86A
No multitasking

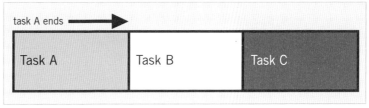

FIGURE 86B
Sequential multitasking

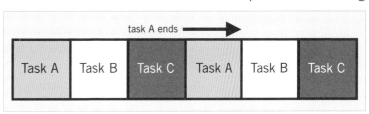

FIGURE 86C
Parallel multi tasking

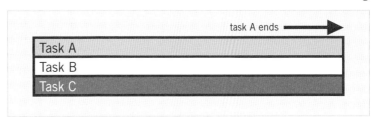

In figure 86A, there is no multitasking. Each task is performed in order, and the end of task 'A' comes $1/3$ of the way through the available time. If 'A' is the task that is on the critical path, this process will deliver the shortest critical path.

In figure 86B, the department works for a while on 'A', then 'B', then 'C', before returning to work on 'A'. This may arise when there are multiple projects, and the priorities are unclear or there are multiple priorities from differing projects. Whatever the cause of the multitasking, in this example Task 'A' now finishes $2/3$ of the way through the available time.

In 86C, there is parallel multitasking. This is very common — the department works on all tasks at once, with none getting priority. In this case, completion of task 'A' takes all the available time.

Multitasking does not deliver any of the three projects in this example faster. Task 'C' is always completed in the same time. However without multitasking, task 'A' is completed more quickly, and if it is on the critical path of a project, the project will suffer fewer delays. This efficiency is in addition to the other problem with multitasking — the lack of focus that comes from switching between jobs. Concentrating on a single task until it is completed will reduce the amount of wasted time and effort that goes into picking up and refamiliarising yourself with a task that has been set aside for a while.

Wasting Safety on parallel tasks

FIGURE 87
Loss of safety with
parallel paths

The final way that safety time can be lost is where tasks are done in parallel. This can be seen in figure 87. Tasks 'B', 'C', 'D' and 'E' are all dependant on task 'A', so cannot start until 'A' is completed. Task 'F' depends on tasks 'B', 'C', 'D' and 'E', so cannot start until all four are completed. Although 'B', 'C' and 'D' are all finished early, the gains in time are meaningless because the next step ('F') cannot start until the late running step 'E' is complete. Although there is more time saved in 'B', 'C' and 'D' than is lost in 'E', in reality savings are lost, and the largest delay is passed onto the project as a whole.

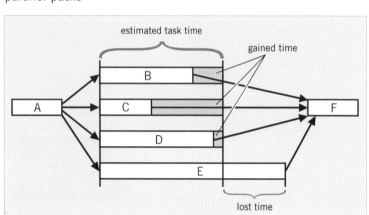

Conclusion

Traditional project management focusses on the achievement of target dates as a way of ensuring that projects meet deadlines. Dates are attached to milestones, and performance is monitored to ensure that intermediate deadlines are met. The project completion date is protected by monitoring every step in the project, and time estimates include large amounts of safety to ensure every step meets its deadline. For the reasons covered, this safety is then lost in a variety of ways, the project runs late, and the final completion date is placed at risk. There must be a better solution!

	Classical Approach	*Critical Chain*
Task duration shown in plan	Durations the estimator is very confident can be achieved	Durations thought to be achievable 50% of the time
Allowances for uncertainty in task duration estimates	Padding within task estimates protects tasks individually. May have contingency reserve at project manager's discretion	Project buffer between end of last scheduled activity and project end date. Buffer sized statistically to protect aggregate project
Shortest project duration controlled by...	Critical Path: sequence of tasks that have zero slack between them from beginning to end	Critical Chain: sequence of tasks that has minimum slack without overloading resources
Project start time	As soon as possible, to maximise time available before deadline	Count backwards project duration (including buffer) from deadline. Hence may not start immediately
Delegated tasks should be finished...	No later than the planned end date (which usually means on planned date or shortly after)	As soon as possible and handed over so that next task can start early
Multitasking	Acceptable (so all tasks done in parallel progress more slowly)	Not done: finish one task so that others can use your outputs, then move on to another
Planning to protect against delay	Risk management plan to prevent risks delaying the project	Risk management plan, and feed buffers and resource buffers, to protect critical chain tasks from variations in input resources and task timing
Management focus	Critical path — which may change when non-critical activities overrun. Hence whole project must be watched	Critical chain — which should not change through the project because of the measures to protect it.
Monitoring metrics	Progress, projected completion date, earned value, schedule performance index, cost performance index etc	Progress and buffer usage

1 From *'The Definitive Guide to Project Management'*, Nokes et al, 2003

Applying critical chain project management

The management of critical chain projects is fundamentally different to traditional project management. There are four main areas of difference: management of safety, floating start times, resource balancing, and monitoring of progress. The differences between the classical approach and the critical chain approach are listed in the table on page 165 but this chapter will cover the main differences in detail.

The management of safety

Safety management in critical chain projects is very simple: stop protecting the tasks, and protect the project.

The Theory of Constraints proposes that in every chain of events there is a constraint — a limiting step — that determines the maximum capacity of the process. In production, it may be a machine. In healthcare improvement projects, it may be a resource such as a critical staff member. In project management, the constraint is the critical chain — the sequence of events that determines the time that the project will take. The Theory of Constraints proposes that we elevate the constraint, ensuring that everything is done to maximise the use of the constraint rather than ensuring that every step in the process is working at a maximum. In Critical Chain project management this translates to ensuring that the critical chain is protected, not the individual tasks in the project.

How to protect the critical chain

Because critical chain project management does not protect individual tasks, there is no need to buffer each task by providing safety. Because we will not monitor on task completion targets, performance is not dependent on completing a task on time. **The only measure we are interested in is the performance of the project overall. The only target we are interested in is the final completion date.**

The fundamental difference between the classical approach and the critical chain approach can be summarised in two steps:

1. Take out the safety from each step

2. Put all the safety where it is needed — at the end of the project

Take out the step safety

This is easy to say, and hard to do. In essence, what is required is to get a 50% completion estimate, not a 90% completion estimate. However, staff used to estimating task durations will be reluctant to accept that their performance will not be measured by meeting the 50% target time. Nokes et al[1] suggest the following approach:

- Ask for a 'confident' estimate (90% likely that the work can be done in this time). *Then* ask for a 50% estimate — the time that the task will be completed in 50% of the times it is done. By asking for both, it is easier to explain the difference between the two estimates and the reason for using the 50% estimate.

FIGURE 88A
Critical chain with 90% esimates

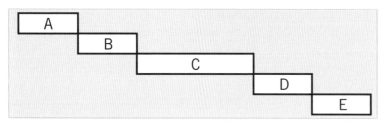

FIGURE 88B
The difference between 50% and 90%

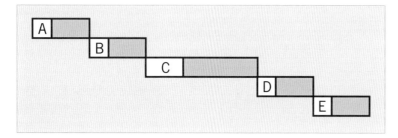

FIGURE 88C
Move all the safety to the end of the project

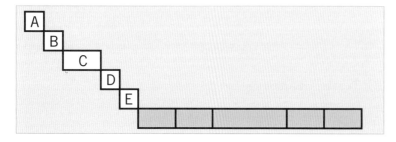

FIGURE 88D
The project buffer reduced to 50%

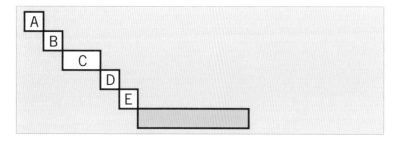

- Get the estimate from someone who knows the task or area well. Try to pick the person who will be actually doing the work, but do not tell them the deadline.

- Get more than one set of estimates if possible.

Once the task estimates are obtained, the excess safety between the 50% and 90% estimates can be removed from each step. The process for transferring the buffer from the steps to the project end is as follows:

- Plan the steps in the project in the normal way (figure 88A)

- Identify the safety that makes up the difference between the 90% estimate and the 50% estimate. This will probably be between 1/2 and 2/3 of the time in each step. (figure 88B)

- Move all the safety to the end of the project. (figure 88C)

- Reduce the safety in the project buffer by 50% (figure 88D).

It is possible to take out half of the project safety because statistically the overruns on each step will now average out. Previously, for the reasons already covered, no step was likely to underrun. Now, with the safety removed from the steps and placed in the project buffer, there is no safety left in the steps to waste.

1 *The Definitive Guide to Project Management.* Nokes et al, 2003

Clearly there is one additional advantage not mentioned so far: the overall project time is reduced significantly. This is a significant feature of critical chain projects; overall project time is usually at least 20% shorter than a project planned in the traditional way, yet the project is more likely to be completed on target or before.

Management of start times

There need to be some rules that work differently for critical chain projects. The first one is the need to start the next step as soon as the previous step is finished. In classical project management, the start time of any step is well known long before it is reached — with the result that it is unlikely that any step will start earlier than planned. In a critical chain project, steps can start early.

This means that the project plan becomes a living document, which may change on a daily basis. It is important that those who are involved in a step about to commence know when they need to be committed; they will need warnings about the upcoming work. It will not be possible to say at the start of the project 'You will be needed from March 23rd for two weeks' but it is possible to say 'You will be needed during March for one week, and we will give you ten days notice of the likely start time, then daily updates from five days before we need you'.

This may seem a problem for planning work in departments, but it should not be. For one thing, the need for prompt start and total commitment is primarily necessary on the critical chain tasks; for another, the pressure to deliver on date target is reduced. In a critical chain project, it is expected that on some tasks (50% in fact) the step end time will be exceeded; all that is asked is that when you start work on a task, it is completed as fast as is possible and handed on to the next step as soon as it is complete.

Monitoring procedures covered later make the communication process easier.

Tasks not on the critical chain

Projects are generally not a linear series of steps, and when the project is planned there will be places where paths diverge and come together. Management of these non-critical paths is also important.

FIGURE 89
Adding feed buffers

Treat each non-critical path as a separate project — calculate the 90% - 50% estimates, move the buffer to the end and reduce by 50%, then add the non-critical path to the overall project plan (figure 89). The feed buffer thus created will absorb the variation in the non-critical path, and protect the critical chain.

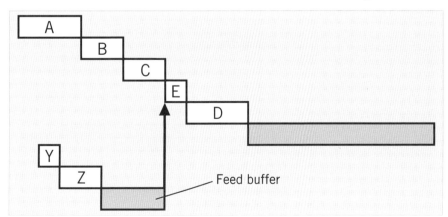

Feed buffer

Resource Balancing

The main difference between managing a critical path and managing a critical chain is in dealing with issues of resource contention.

Often projects will use specific resources in more then one place. For example, production of a series of posters and displays may be organised by differing groups of people, but all arrive at the print unit at the same time. If the time allocation for printing has been based on one task arriving, several will cause the task to overrun significantly. This is a common problem in classical project management, and is one reason why critical tasks take longer than the 50% estimate of time. The problem is made worse if the overloaded department then uses multitasking to manage the overload.

Figure 90A shows a project where several strands of work come together into step 'R'. The critical path for this project is 'P-Q-G-H-I-R', which represents the longest single chain of events.

Figure 90B shows the same project, but with the steps undertaken by a common resource coloured. Steps 'Q', 'C', 'F', 'L' and 'O' are all performed by the same person. Clearly there is a problem meeting the deadline for step 'R' as four of the preceding five steps are done by the same person.

Figure 90C shows the same project with the contentions resolved. Now there is no time where the common resource is working on more than one step, however the critical path time has increased. In order to re-arrange the steps to avoid contentions, extra time has had to be allowed between steps 'Q' and 'G'.

Figure 90D shows the critical chain overlaid with a dotted line. The critical path ('P-Q-G-H-I-R') is still the longest sequence of events, and it has a period of delay built in as a result of the resource contention resolution. However, the critical chain ('P-Q-O-L-C-F-R') is the series of tasks which determine the timing of the overall project. It is this series of timings that is required to determine the project buffer, and these are the events that will need monitoring to ensure that the final deadline is met.

Progress Monitoring

There are many ways to monitor traditional projects. Performance to time is usually managed by comparing what proportion of work has been done on tasks to date, comparing dates when milestones were achieved with the target dates for those milestones, and measuring how far out the final completion date has been pushed.

Progress monitoring in a critical chain project is much simpler. There are two basic measures: how far through is the project, and how much of the final buffer has been utilised. Additionally, you need to measure feed buffer usage for non-critical paths of work underway.

Proportion of project completed

As the project progresses the proportion of the project complete is expressed as a simple percentage:

$$\frac{\text{Work Done}}{\text{Total amount of work}}$$

It is important to measure the total amount of work correctly — if several tasks have overrun, the total amount of work is not the same as the original estimate. Asking people to estimate simply how far they are through the task will give a different estimate to "How many more days will it be until the task is complete?"

The equation should read:

$$\frac{\text{Work Done}}{(\text{Work done} + \text{Work still to do})}$$

expressed as a percentage.

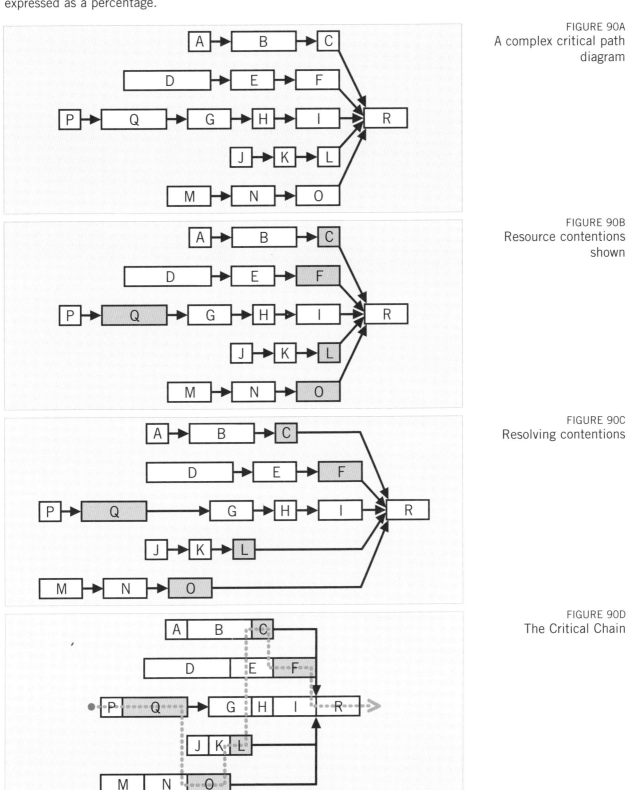

FIGURE 90A
A complex critical path diagram

FIGURE 90B
Resource contentions shown

FIGURE 90C
Resolving contentions

FIGURE 90D
The Critical Chain

Final Buffer utilisation

The key measure for whether the project is on track is the amount of the final buffer that has been used. All variation in performance is transferred to this buffer, and monitoring is a simple process of determining how much of the buffer is used at a certain point in time.

The proportion of buffer use is related to the amount of the total project completed. A project that is 10% complete and has used 50% of the buffer is far more at risk than one that is 90% complete and has used 80% of the buffer. Accordingly, the best way to represent buffer use is as a run chart with bands of risk (figure 91).

Where less than 1/3 of the buffer has been used, the project is on track (green). Where less than 2/3 is used, the project is at risk and planning should be undertaken to resolve problems that have arisen (amber). There is no need to take action at this stage, just to prepare plans.

Where over two thirds of the buffer is used, the project is in severe risk and the plans previously determined must be put in place.

In the white zone, the proportion of the buffer used is less than would be expected, and it is likely that the project will end early. In the black zone, all the buffer has been used and it is likely that the project will end late.

Feeder chain buffers can be monitored in the same way. In the case of feed buffers which run into the black zone, the excess buffer use must be transferred to the project buffer, as exceeding the feed buffer will impact on the critical chain. Unfortunately, time saved (the feed buffer is in the white zone) does not correspondingly reduce the project buffer.

Monitoring project costs

This approach to reporting time management can also be used to monitor project budgets and costs. Rather than allowing contingency in each budget item, estimate budgets as 50% likelihood that they will not be exceeded. Allow contingency as a 'cost buffer' and manage budget performance as proportion of cost buffer used. Although cost is not quite the same as time (savings are not as likely to be lost in budget items as time is in task items), using a consistent reporting methodology does have advantages.

FIGURE 91
Project buffer monitoring

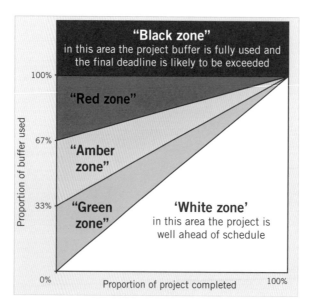

Managing critical chain in a classical environment

Critical chain project management is a relatively new approach to project management, and only a minority of NHS Trusts use the approach. In most Trusts, project management uses traditional approaches, typically PRINCE2 methodology.

Traditional methodology exists to improve project success, and it does this through three key features. These features need to be present in a critical chain approach, just in a slightly different form.

1. A clear project scope document

All projects include some form of statement of scope. In PRINCE2, a Project Initiation Document (PID) is the first document produced, and critical chain projects also need a PID. The importance of the PID is to describe what is in, what is out, and who is involved.

What is in and what is out, the scope of the project, are essential to prevent 'scope creep', where the goal of the project changes over time. Scope creep is a sure way to fail to meet deadlines and deliver the original purpose of the project, and having a clear written definition of the scope of the project from the start will prevent this happening.

It is also important to make clear from the start who is involved in the project. Projects consume resources and time, and these must be stated in the PID. The sponsors and customers of the project should also be included in the PID, so that processes are clear for changing the PID if it becomes necessary.

Traditional PID structures such as PRINCE2 templates will work perfectly well with critical chain project management.

2. A clear project plan

The project plan for PRINCE2 will include a Gantt chart, with task times, sequencing and milestone dates. The critical path will be clear from the plan.

The project plan for critical chain will also include a Gantt chart, with 50% task time estimates and buffers clearly indicated. The project buffer, feed chain buffers, and resource buffers (buffers to protect access to essential resources) should be clearly shown. There may be milestones marked, but these should not be deadline milestones. The Gantt chart must also contain constraint resolution, and the critical chain will be clear. The project plan may look very different to the conventional plan, and it will be important to explain why buffers exist, and why they cannot be trimmed arbitrarily.

3. Reporting mechanisms

What to report and to whom? Reporting progress is essential for communication within the team and the wider customer group, as well as to those managing and sponsoring the project. Writing a regular report is also valuable to ensure that the project manager focusses on the project status on a regular basis.

PRINCE2 reporting focusses on achievement of milestone dates, and progress along the Gantt chart. Critical chain project reporting focusses on the proportion of the project completed, and the proportion of the project buffer used. These concepts are very different, and if reports are going to people unfamiliar with critical chain, some work will be necessary to explain what the reports mean.

Reports will normally go to some form of board or steering group, and this group, which will have oversight responsibilities for the project, must understand that the project is being managed in a different fashion. Providing copies of this chapter, the critical chain presentation on the NLIAH website, or the books listed in Chapter 10 may help in explaining the concepts to those unfamiliar with the Theory of Constraints. The NLIAH has developed a quick critical chain game that can be used in groups to get the basic concepts across.

Conclusion

Project management is essential if projects are to succeed, and if the NHS is to improve, projects must succeed at a higher rate than in the past. Traditional methods of managing projects have not been as successful as desired and in part this is due to some flawed principles involved in traditional project management methodology. Simply increasing the amount of documentation, and the detail in reporting, with more dates, more intermediate milestones and more sanctions, will not address the fundamental flaws in traditional project management. Doing the same thing over and over in more detail and expecting to get a different result is a sign of muddled thinking.

Critical chain is a powerful way of managing projects using the core principles of Goldratt's Theory of Constraints. It addresses many of the problems of traditional project management, yet contains the essentials of good planning and reporting. More importantly, it works. It delivers projects faster, at less cost, and more reliably.

It works.

Integrated Care Pathways

An Integrated Care Pathway (ICP) is a document that describes a process within Health and Social Care. An ICP is not a process map; this is a misconception. ICP is a tool and a concept, which embeds guidelines, protocols and locally agreed evidence-based patient-centred best practice, into everyday use for the individual patient. Uniquely to ICPs, they record deviations from planned care in the form of 'variances'.

The term 'Care Pathway' is often misused and there are many so called 'care pathways' being developed and implemented across Wales with no uniformity. One objective of the 'Innovations in Care Integrated Care Pathway programme', which ran in 2003, was to clarify the standards that make up an Integrated Care Pathway.

FIGURE 92
What is an Integrated
Care Pathway?

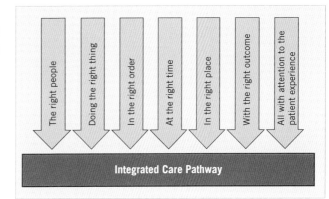

THE GOLD STANDARD FOR DEVELOPMENT FOR INTEGRATED CARE PATHWAYS AS AGREED BY THE INTEGRATED CARE PATHWAY NETWORK 2003

An Integrated Care Pathway is anticipated care placed in an appropriate time frame, written and agreed by a multidisciplinary team. It has locally agreed standards based on evidence where available to help a patient with a specific condition or diagnosis move progressively through the clinical experience.
It forms part or all of the clinical record, documenting the care given.
It facilitates and demonstrates continuous quality improvement. It includes patient milestones and clinical interventions noted on the day or stage that they are expected to occur. It will include all of the following standards or show evidence that it is working towards meeting these standards:
- Multidisciplinary
- Cross Boundaries
- Single Documentation
- Standard Format
- Use exception reporting
- Outcome orientated
- Variance analysis
- Built in audit
- Patient/user involvement
- Evidence based
- Monitoring of the utilisation

Innovations in Care, Welsh Assembly Government 2003

The ICP is structured around the 'variance tracking tool' and it describes a process for a discreet element of care i.e. primary care, admission, acute care, rehabilitation, discharge etc. These elements build together to construct a unique journey for each individual patient according to their need based on professional judgement. It sets out anticipated outcomes that are locally agreed and reflect a patient-centred, multi-disciplinary, multi-agency approach. It must be noted that although certain elements of care can be entirely 'unidisciplinary', they cannot be constructed without the knowledge and input of the whole multidisciplinary team.

ICPs should be based on evidence where the evidence is available. Whilst it may take some time to reach the standard that all ICPs are evidence based, this should be the goal. However, lack of agreement on evidence based standards for a condition, or lack of national standards, should not be seen as a barrier to ICP development. As a first step, internal best practice should be adopted as the ICP standard.

ICPs should be developed by a multidisciplinary team and should deal with all aspects of patient care. Existing individual speciality or professionally based ICPs (e.g. nursing, medical and allied health professional notes) and all other documentation relating to the patient's care, should be incorporated into the ICP document and be available to all professionals involved in the patient's care. This is essential to ensure patient focused care.

ICPs are intended to be a guide to providing care for the patient and their family. The multidisciplinary document can replace existing patient notes for this period of care. Professionals are encouraged to exercise their own professional judgement. However, any alteration to the practice identified within the ICP must be recorded as a variance. If appropriate, patients can come off the ICP.

The ICP document becomes all or part of the contemporaneous patient/client record. Completed activities, outcomes and variations between planned and actual care are recorded at the point of delivery.

Wherever possible, reporting on ICPs should be by exception, with agreed standards incorporated into the ICP. Entries on to the ICP document should be either initialled by the professional responsible for that element of care to confirm that the expected standard is met or details should be given of why/where the standard has not been met. All ICPs will contain an 'identification sheet' where all professionals involved in a patient's care can log their initials and their full name and designation.

ICPs should focus on outcomes. Standards should be set for patients progressing through their care journey and achieving key milestones. This allows variations in inputs to be correlated with exceptions in outcomes to determine how care or the ICP can be improved.

A stakeholder is anyone who may have an interest in the ICP or its outcomes. Stakeholders may therefore be identified under two categories: those for whom a consultation exercise would be appropriate (external stakeholders) and those who need to be directly involved in the development of the ICP (internal stakeholders). Stakeholders require a clear mechanism through which they can ask questions, feedback and give ideas or express concerns. It is better to address these issues early in the process than to wait until the implementation stage, when the ICP itself could be undermined.

ICP development should involve patients where appropriate by the use of tools mentioned later in the guide. Patient representatives can also be involved where possible within the bounds of confidentiality, in variance analysis and ICP development. (See figure 93)

FIGURE 93
External and Internal
Stakeholders

EXTERNAL AND INTERNAL STAKEHOLDERS

Indirectly Involved
- Trust Boards
- Medical Advisory Committee
- Nursing Advisory Group
- Social Services
- Voluntary associations

Directly involved
- User, e.g. Patient, Carers, Advocacy services
- ICP project team staff
- Referrers
- Relevant Departments e.g. Clinical Governance, IM&T
- Other Agencies
- Specialist Services
- Other Organisations
- The Multi Disciplinary Teams
- Primary Care

ICP Process Mapping

As ICPs are tools for improving care delivered to patients, then it follows, that in order to make improvements, a firm understanding of what is actually happening is required and this is best done through a process mapping exercise. The patient journey must be captured, understood and analysed by the whole clinical team, key stakeholders and patients.

From this position the team can begin to determine how the process mapping information can be translated into the first draft of the ICP.

ICP Contents

ICPs should contain:

- Activities — These are the planned elements of care contained in the process. They are based on evidence based best practice (EBBP)

- Detail — Any tools or descriptions already required in the case notes, including observations, fluid balance charts, demographic details etc

- Outcomes — These can range from clinical outcomes (tests etc) to process outcomes (e.g. standards achieved against targets) and may include patient or staff outcomes.

- Variance Tracking — The unique element of an ICP that allows planned and actual care to be compared, leading to continuous improvement of practice.

The clinical content of an ICP cannot be dictated; this will be determined by the team with expertise in managing that particular group of patients for whom the document is designed.

Variance Tracking

ICPs as mentioned offer a structure for care delivery, they do not replace or compromise individual practitioner's clinical judgement or decision making. They are not a substitute for clinical judgement.

Not all patients will follow a predicable ICP. Any professional may and should deviate from the ICP provided they have a valid reason and rationale for doing so; the intent is for clinical freedom to be exercised according to individual patient need. This is known as a 'variance'.

Variances occur when what is expected to happen does not. Variances are then recorded by the professional, noting why the decision was made and what remedial or alternative action, was or is to be taken (ICPUS[1]). This is known as 'variance tracking'.

The method by which variances are documented may vary from organisation to organisation. However variance tracking is undertaken within individual organisations, Shuttleworth[2] discusses the vital components necessary for structured variance tracking to ensure that all required variances in care are monitored and analysed. She suggests that the method used should be quick, intuitive, accessible, meaningful, part of normal routine record keeping and clearly linked to the relevant activity by a unique identifier. It should not involve the practitioner in time wasting duplication, searching out tracking sheets and working out how to complete them or having to describe, in longhand, the activity in question.

Reasons for deviation from the ICP will be noted within the documentation and this may be due to individual clinical judgement, operational or systems failure, time lapses, blockages in the system or patient choice. When variance tracking has been audited, trends can be easily identified. Trends can help to manage clinical risk and allow for the evaluation of care provided through the ICP. This information can then be fed back to the individual clinical teams to enable them to establish a clear picture of what is happening, which may in turn, highlight training or education deficits or a need to revisit and amend the ICP.

ICP Development — The Four Step Model

The development of ICPs is by no means simple but the process can be streamlined by adopting a structured approach. The ICP development structure takes the form of four meetings in which particular elements are covered. Before every, preparatory work will need to be conducted by the key members of the development team to create a platform from which to base the agenda of the following meeting. Figure 94 explains the four step model in brief. Figure 95, starting on page 182, provides more detail of each step in the process.

1 *ICP users Scotland*, 2003
www.icpus.ukprofessionals.com

2 *NT Protocol based care.*
Shuttleworth A (ED), 2003
emap healthcare

FIGURE 94
The 'Four Step'
development model
in brief

STEP 1

Meeting 1 Preparation

1.1 *Before the first meeting:* Collect baseline data on patient/condition on which the ICP will focus

1.2 Explain to the team what an ICP is and have a copy of an extant ICP of the specialty available

1.3 Develop a high level patient flow process map

1.4 Identify where the ICP will start and finish

1.5 Identify the stages of care in the ICP

1.6 Identify the patient discharge criteria

1.7 Identify the perceived problems with the current care

STEP 2

Meeting 2 Preparation

2.1 *Before Meeting 2:* Each member of the team to confirm discharge criteria with wider colleague circle and to do the same for the perceived problems with the current care

2.2 Confirm perceived problems with the current care

2.3 Decide how to identify if perceived problems really 'are' problems

2.4 Develop a plan for collecting sample data to identify if perceived problems really 'are' problems

2.5 Develop an initial list of 'ultimate patient outcomes' that the ICP needs to focus on

STEP 3

Meeting 3 Preparation

3.1 *Before Meeting 3:* Each professional within the team to identify their particular areas of responsibility within each stage of the ICP

3.2 Professionals to present back to the team their particular areas of responsibility

3.3 Presentation of the confirmed problems with the current care

3.4 Identify how to minimise the problems

3.5 Determine the criteria patients must meet to pass through the discreet stages of the ICP

STEP 4

Meeting 4 Preparation

4.1 Each member to develop a final list of individual professionals' inputs and patient outcomes/expectations

4.2 One member to develop draft clinical and patient version of ICP and distribute

4.3 Review the draft ICP and agree final amendments

4.4 Identify ICP and team's ability to deliver on agreed outcomes

4.5 Develop a plan for the ICP pilot phase

4.6 Set up a variance tracking database

Once the ICP has been developed it is very important to ensure that the momentum for using the ICP is maintained. This can be supported by organising a post-pilot review meeting which will identify what problems were encountered during the ICP implementation phase. During this meeting, a team will be established to regularly review the ICP and any variances. Subsequently, the ICP review team should meet regularly and if necessary establish small working parties to look at particular trends detected by variance tracking and identify whether processes or care requires improvement.

ICP Implementation & Change

As with any process of change, careful preparation needs to be made for the implementation of the ICP. This preparation begins sometime before the ICP documentation is ready for use, when the wider clinical team need to be made aware of the developments that are taking place. The appearance of the ICP in the clinical area should not come as a shock!

Below is a guide to the ICP implementation process:

- Inform staff in the area prior to the launch date — circulate copies of the ICP so they are familiar with the layout. Notices can be used to increase awareness.
- Arrange training sessions for all staff who will come into contact with the ICP — this will involve going through a copy of the documentation, explaining its purpose and how it should be completed, especially the recording of variances.
- Pilot the ICP for a set period of time or for a set number of cases: this will depend on the patient group for whom the ICP has been developed
- Ensure that copies of the ICP are kept in an accessible place and that staff know where to find them (e.g. in a clearly labeled open box).
- Put a 'comments/communication sheet' near the spare copies of the ICP in the Clinical area so any queries, comments or issues can be noted.

Remember when piloting/implementing the ICP, there must be....
- support for local clinical leads to deliver ICP training to pilot teams
- senior staff support of each local ICP for the first week of running
- maintenance of the high profile of the ICP throughout the pilot period
- re-launch the updated ICP — including publicity and feedback from pilot
- remove pilot versions and replace with the updated version
- NB: If you number the pilot copies, you will know which ones are missing
- Long-term implementation. Remember:
- There must be a regular variance tracking feedback session incorporated into routine educational/team sessions. It is this that will prevent the 'fizzling out' syndrome that projects are prone to.

Evaluation the ICP

Evaluation of the ICP is very much an ongoing process and all ICPs should be viewed as 'living documents'. After the pilot phase, things tend to settle down as the new version is launched for a longer period of time. The ICP is a dynamic tool which needs to be reviewed and amended as part of the ongoing audit process — the frequency of review depends on the variances recorded. Variance recording allows any deviation from the expected plan of care to be monitored to ensure that the ICP continues to meet the needs of the patient group it was designed for and to be amended to reflect the latest developments in evidence based best practice.

When evaluating the ICP, the following should be considered:

- **Completion of the ICP** — is it being used in all appropriate cases? How is it being completed? What information is being omitted? Are staff using conventional record keeping in addition/instead of the ICP?
- **Types of Variances Recorded** — have any been recorded, if so are they appropriate? Is it clear that staff know what variances are and how to record them?
- **Staff satisfaction** — a generic questionnaire which may be available from your local Trust Care ICP Manager.

This chapter is a summary extracted from *A Guide to Good Practice: Integrated Care Pathways* Published by the NLIAH, 2005

FIGURE 95
The 'Four Step'
process in detail
(continued on
next pages)

The Four Step Model: Sub-Step Descriptions/Examples

Step 1		Explanation
1.1	**Before the first meeting:** Collect baseline data on patient/condition on which the ICP will focus	Once you have decided what ICP to develop and what patients group to focus on, you need to gather data to inform the ICP such as ALOS, type of admission, discharge destination, date of surgery etc. This information will illustrate the variation within current practice attributable to either the patient or clinical care
1.2	Explain to the team what an ICP is and have a copy of an extant ICP of the specialty available	Everyone who will be expected to use the ICP needs to know what it is. Use the ICP to see what others are doing and to identify how your ICP will need to be different
1.3	Develop a high level patient flow process map	Using process mapping methodology, gather the relevant people into a room and develop your high level process map. This is the perfect opportunity to give professionals a chance to see the current process from the patients' perspective and take out steps which do not add value to patient care
1.4	Identify where the ICP will start and finish	The ICP has to have a clear beginning and end. This may be the moment patients enter the GP surgery to entering the hospital or entering ITU to discharge. It is easier to develop ICP within one organisation rather than to develop across organisational boundaries but it is feasible to do so.
1.5	Identify the stages of care in the ICP	Within an ICP, there will be discreet stages of care e.g., assessment, post surgical, discharge. Identify these stages so that the ICP development is more focused and does not appear so daunting
1.6	Identify the patient discharge criteria	From the outset, you need to have clear ideas about what the patient discharge criteria are. Identifying the discharge destination and working back can assist in identifying discharge criteria. Criteria should include physical, domestic, social and transport planning, e.g. is the patient happy to go home, does the patient have transport to take them home
1.7	Identify the perceived problems with the current care	It is likely that within the current system there are problems. Identify what you think these problems are

Step 2		Explanation
2.1	**Before Meeting 2:** Each member of the team to confirm discharge criteria with wider colleague circle and to do the same for the perceived problems with the current care	After the first meeting, all the members need to go away and talk to their specialty colleagues to get a consensus on whether the discharge criteria and the perceived problems which the group has come up with are suitable and actually perceived
2.2	Confirm perceived problems with the current care	In the team, you need to discuss the perceived problems as discussed and agreed in your specialty areas
2.3/2.4	Decide how to identify if perceived problems really 'are' problems and develop a plan for collecting sample data to identify if perceived problems really 'are' problems	Once you have a list of perceived problems, you need to develop a plan to identify whether they really are problems. This will probably involve collecting data from notes or developing a data collection exercise to run for a few weeks. Keep the data collection exercise small, e.g. medical records of the last 10 admitted patients
2.5	Develop an initial list of 'ultimate patient outcomes' that the ICP needs to focus on	Based on the variations in care (linked to 1.1) and perceived problems (linked to 1.7, 2.3, 2.4), identify the best practice patient focused aims which the ICP needs to focus on, e.g. 70% of patients can go home in 3 days

Step 3		
		Explanation
3.1	**Before Meeting 3:** Each professional within the team to identify their particular areas of responsibility within each stage of the ICP	Linking to 1.5, the members of the group now need to look in detail at the sections now need to look in detail at the sections within the ICP which are particularly pertinent to them and for which they have responsibility, such as nursing, clerking, discharge. The group needs to refer to the best practice evidence available and record relevant references.
3.2	Professionals to present back to the team their particular areas of responsibility	Once members of the team have had an opportunity to discuss their responsibilities with specialty colleagues, these findings need to be fed back to the team
3.3	Presentation of the confirmed problems with the current care	The team needs to discuss the original perceived problems, as previously discussed with colleagues, in light of the data collection exercise. (linked to 3.1) A list of confirmed actual problems needs to be drawn up.
3.4	Identify how to minimise the problems	The group needs to confirm that the actual problems which can not be addressed prior to the ICP implementation, will be addresses within the ICP plan of care. It may be necessary to develop new strategies in the plan to address the problems e.g. add in additional care plan for patients with diabetes
3.5	Determine the criteria patients must meet to pass through the discreet stages of the ICP	Determine the interim goals the patient needs to attain to pass through the discreet stages within the ICP. This may mean 'patient is able to walk unaided' and therefore can pass to the discharge section

Step 4		Explanation
4.1	**Before Meeting 4:** Each member to develop a final list of individual professionals' inputs and patient outcomes/ expectations	The draft lists of patient outcomes and staff responsibilities need to be forwarded to the member for the team collating the information
4.2	**Before Meeting 4:** One member to develop draft clinical and patient version of ICP and distribute	One member of the team needs to put all of the information together and write the draft ICP. ICPs need to focus on patient outcomes. Draw up a draft list of these outcomes, e.g. rather than having an aim of 'nurse supports patient to sit in chair', think about 'patient is able to sit in chair with support'. The ICP is not about the nurse but the patient. If your organisation has decided to adopt a patient version of the ICP, this would also be the time to write a draft version
4.3	Review the draft ICP and agree final amendments	In the final meeting, the team needs to go through the draft ICP and agree the final version. If this does not happen now, there is a danger that the ICP will continue to be modified and amended and never become 'live'
4.4	Identify ICP and team's ability to deliver on agreed outcomes	The group needs to confirm that the care plan within the ICP does minimise actual problems (linking to 3.4, 3.5) and maximises the ICP and the clinical teams' ability to deliver on the ICPs patient focused aims (linked to 2.5)
4.5	Develop a plan for the ICP pilot phase	The pilot phase needs to be planned. You need to decide who will conduct the initial training, it is useful to have a combination of training styles such as seminars, one-to-one meetings etc. Rather than focusing on a specified time to conduct the pilot, it will be more useful to identify a specific number of ICPs/patients, maybe 10.
4.6	Set up a variance tracking database	In order to make the best use of the variances, you need to develop a variance tracking database. This may be developed by your department, trust or may be a manual system. NLIAH has a database which you may find useful to use. The best analysis will be gained by collecting variance data from patients at the time that the variance occurs, rather than in retrospect; this minimises work and the possibility of data being lost or forgotten. It is important that variance data is collected for each patient otherwise the team will not gain adequate feedback on what is happening with the guidelines in the pathways.

Having the tools and techniques for change does not make change happen. The human elements in the change process must also be taken into account. The next few chapters deal with those human problems of change and leadership.

Key Points:

- There are certain predictable conditions that will help a change process succeed

- Management cultures and leadership styles are essential determinants of success or failure

- Management of how staff 'feel' about change is also central to success

- PDSA cycles give us a model for achieving change in challenging environments

- Feedback mechanisms can also bring about change

Leadership, culture and managing change

9

Previous chapters have covered analysis tools. But analysis is not enough. Analysis without action is an academic exercise. This chapter covers some basic tools for implementation of change.

Leadership and Culture
Good leadership in a change environment is one of the key determinants of success. The elements of a successful change programme and leadership styles for change are covered here.

The human dimensions
Change happens when people want change to happen. Taking the staff and patients along with you on the change process is essential.

PDSA cycles: A model for improvement
The use of PDSA cycles as a mechanism for delivering change has revolutionised the change process in England, Wales and the United States where the technique was first developed.

GP feedback systems
The use of access protocols in primary care is a common way of trying to reduce demand on secondary care services. NLIAH recommends an alternative to access protocols, the use of active feedback to GPs.

CARDIFF AND VALE NHS TRUST
Using 'Plan Do Study Act' cycles in Endoscopy

Demand and Capacity principles are being applied to Endoscopy services at the University Hospital of Wales. Detailed process-mapping at multi-disciplinary workshops identified opportunities to improve patient preparation prior to the endoscopy examination as a means of increasing the number of patients who attend.

The team planned a PDSA cycle by selecting an Endoscopy list for non-urgent patients, and training a senior nurse to carry out telephone pre-admission assessment of patients. Data collected included changes in patient attendance rates and the time taken to assess the patient with and without the service.

On completion of the PDSA cycle the nurse-led pre-admission service was shown to have achieved a reduction in patients' non-attendanc or cancellation rate from 18% to 6%, which if made available to all patients, could increase patient attendances by up to 500 per year.

Leadership and culture

What makes individual programmes successful? This chapter reviews the evidence for change programmes, and goes on to look at how the culture of an organisation or groups within organisations can make change hard work. Finally, it looks at leadership styles which are most likely to provide a culture which favours change.

Running a successful change programme — Process issues

Trisha Greenhalgh and colleagues reviewed 1000 research papers to find the attributes of an innovation which encourage its uptake[1]. They are:

Relative Advantage: There must be evidence that the innovation can improve things.

Low Complexity: It should be possible to understand and publicise the innovation simply or broken down into simple parts.

Compatibility: The change needs to be compatible with how people work and with their values.

Trialability: It should be possible to try out the innovation without making full commitment.

Observability: Improvements can be associated with the innovation.

Capacity for Reinvention: It must be possible to adapt the innovation to the individual needs of the organisation.

These findings reinforce the usefulness of PDSA cycles: planning a change, carrying out the change, studying and evaluating the outcome and further fine-tuning the innovation.

Greenhalgh has also observed that few changes in health services conform to these principles. Change is often driven by policy or directives where relative advantage may not be obvious, complexity is high and trialability poor. That doesn't mean that such changes are impossible to implement or worthless. Instead Greenhalgh's checklist provides a guide for how implementation must be managed. In the case of an NLIAH programme, the development work will include gathering of evidence of relative advantage. For each site, and for each team involved on each site, the work which must follow includes:

- Mapping the expected gains for this location.

- Translating the overall programme into the elements which are visible to each team.

1 Greenhalgh and MacFarlane in *Health Management* Volume 8 Number 4, 2004

■ Ensuring that new work systems are merged with those that exist and that staff have direct input in design.

■ Agreeing a strategy for monitoring implementation within each department, if necessary using proxy measures

■ Responding flexibly to requests which build on the innovation within the local context.

This checklist is equally applicable to, for example, implementing an NSF or applying a new Medicines Management policy. If all this seems like too much work, the evidence is that if change is not managed in this way it will fail. The consequences of a failed change are wasted resources and less likelihood of co-operation next time. Time spent in preparation and planning is not wasted.

Running a successful change programme — People Issues
Gollop[1] and colleagues studied doctors' and managers' scepticism and resistance to two service improvement programmes in England: The National Booking Programme and the Cancer Services Collaborative. Almost all doctors were sceptical, at least to start with. Managers were less so. The reasons for scepticism included:

■ Concern about national targets being given more priority than local service improvement.

■ Perception of top-down, government led approach.

■ Belief that political targets were transient.

■ Disagreement with the priority given to the programme.

■ Belief that changes to booking systems were trivial.

■ Personal reasons like loss of power, fear of change, disruption of cherished systems.

Overcoming this scepticism is hard work. The successful strategies are:

■ Hearing messages from peers.

■ Seeing practical illustrative examples.

■ Involvement in practical work, especially process mapping.

■ Time, persuasion, PERSISTENCE.

Techniques which challenge doubts and which remove uncertainty of the change are also helpful. Site visits to centres which have implemented the change may serve a number of these purposes as do learning sets and email groups. It is essential that such exercises remain positive — 'Finding ways that we can do it' — rather than negative — 'supporting one another in the belief that we cannot cope.'

Organisational Culture
As organisations become quality driven they pass through three stages.

1 *Influencing sceptical staff to become supporters of service improvement.* Gollop et al, 2004

When an organisation is at the early stages of service improvement, there will be some (hopefully many) spontaneous innovations that seek to improve services. In a typical NHS organisation, the complexity of operation and high educational needs of staff will mean that there are many such innovations occurring all the time. Each innovation will be 'owned' by its originator and, in that sense, well accepted. It may not spread quickly or at all and it may not be sustained.

At the next stage of development, organisations undertake quality improvement programmes which can deliver specific goals and targets. The programmes also encourage better use of information, spread of quality improvement expertise and can enlist more staff to the cause of service improvement. Their downside is that they are expensive and the support for change may remain fragile. They are also rather top-down: the drive for and the context of the programme are usually from 'the centre'.

Quality improvement will only be achieved when it is central to the organisation. The Chief Executive must be the quality champion for the organisation. Karl Weick described the attributes of an organisation whose work is highly reliable:

- A preoccupation with failure.

- Sensitivity to operations.

- Reluctance to simplify interpretations.

- Deference to expertise.

- Commitment to resilience.

While almost everyone who works in the NHS and Social Services is working hard and doing their best, few organisations have reached this third stage.

The remainder of this chapter looks at cultural reasons which inhibit or slow change and the role of leadership.

Inhibitors of quality improvement

Personal Reasons

Issuing an instruction or protocol is not always an effective way of changing a person's working practice. In fact, it may produce inventive resistance. That is because actions are not only driven by logic and instructions. The so called 'Galileo Reality Model' relates behaviour and results to the needs of an individual (see figure 96).

FIGURE 96
The Galileo Reality Model

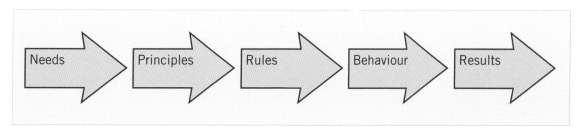

FIGURE 97
Four needs of an
individual

A person's needs are a balance between the need to live, the need to be loved, the need to feel important or valued and the need for variety (see figure 97).

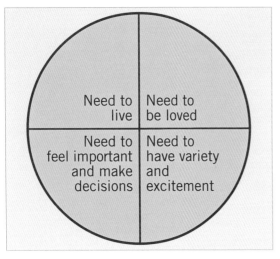

When we achieve balance or equilibrium, our needs guide the formation of our principles or values. They in turn drive our rules on what we do and hence our behaviour.

An external force may make us change our behaviour by threatening our needs. It is easy to see how a protocol or NSF could be threatening in this way. It may threaten variety, suppress individuality and worth. It may even threaten to take away aspects of someone's work and appear to threaten their livelihood.

A change agent or manager's role is to understand and minimise these threats. Confrontations are extremely damaging. Often, vehement resistance to a change may mask the actual threat.

Organisational Complacency

John Kotter[1] refers to too much complacency in an organisation. If an organisation prides itself on being successful it may not share knowledge with others and not be prepared to learn. In turn, it may have a false view of its prowess and the reasons for its good reputation may be past or superficial.

A sense of urgency can only be created by genuine self criticism and a focus on getting it right.

Destructive Management Culture

In contrast to complacency, some organisations institutionalise non-achievement through the conversations between managers. Rather like 'the games people play' these conversations are actually circular and mask what is really going on. This game might be called 'It's good here isn't it?' and consists of a merry nihilism where people reinforce the message that good things do not happen in the organisation, so why try?

Jim Clemmer[2] talks about another destructive culture as 'Sniping, stones and snowballs.' Team members poke fun at one another to raise the laughter index but too often slip below good clean fun. If someone gets hurt, the offender will say 'I was only joking.'

The only effective way of dealing with these behaviours is to keep them in check. They must be challenged, preferably gently.

Not owning the problem

Don Berwick[3] describes two Japanese words: Taseki and Jiseki. Taseki means 'the burden is yours' and is about passing the buck. When an organisation appears to be doing badly, the first response is 'the data are wrong, there's no problem'.

The next line of defence is to admit there is a problem but to disown it, 'Yes our service is poor but we are in the lower quartile of professional staff per inpatient day'. 'Those standards do not reflect our urban setting/our rural setting'. Gollop[4] et al describes a clinician's reaction to the cancer services

1 *Leading Change.* Kotter, 1996

2 *The Leader's digest: Timeless Principles for Team and Organisational Success.* Clemmer, 2003

3 *Improvement, trust and the healthcare workforce.* Berwick, 2003, in Quality and Safety in Healthcare volume 12 supplement 1

4 *Influencing sceptical staff to become supporters of service improvement.* Gollop et al 2004 in Quality and Safety in Healthcare volume 13 number 2

collaborative. "One of my colleague's first responses was to start doing an audit to show that all his 'stone' patients were suffering as a result of this emphasis on cancer work".

All of these reactions signify that no effort will be put into service improvement. Perceived lack of resources is probably one of the most common issues. It can even be justified with an implied logic: "If we make the best of what we've got, we will weaken our strategic case for more resources".

Berwick makes the point that this kind of culture is most likely in a culture of 'Taylorism' — after Frederick Taylor, a 19th-20th century industrialist and author. Taylorism is epitomised by a lack of trust in the workforce and a command/control regime. The joke attributed to Taylor is that when asked how many people worked in his factory he said "about half". It is a self-fulfilling prophecy.

The alternative, jiseki, is about ownership of the problem. It is a harder route than taseki and requires perseverance. As Berwick says, from the point of view of jiseki, blaming cost constraints, the environment, the regulators or anybody else is not an acceptable plan.

The effective strategy is to encourage and invest in an imaginative workforce.

Dominant Professional Cultures

The provision of high quality services and the impetus constantly to improve required connection between clinical decisions and resources, accountability, effective systems and efficient teamworking. Pieter Degeling[1] and colleagues studied these values in doctors, nurses and managers in four countries including Wales. The professional groups behaved remarkably consistently regardless of their country. Doctors opposed all four of the principles of resource awareness, accountability, systematisation and multidisciplinary teams. Nurse managers and general managers, on the other hand, supported or were equivocal about all four.

Clinician idiosyncrasy is often excused on the basis that it reflects patient preference. However, it is seldom the case that patients are given sufficient information to make real choices. An analogy can be drawn between doctors and airline pilots. Airline passengers are given large amounts of information and can select between routes, dates, times and levels of quantity. The reliability of airline flights is dependable. Few people will care who is the pilot but no-one doubts his or her professionalism.

Rene Amalberti[2], himself a doctor working in the aerospace industry, says that if medical services are to have reliability and safety which approach those of other industries, there is a:

▪ Need to place limits on the discretion of workers.

▪ Need to reduce worker autonomy.

▪ Need to transition from craftsmanship attitude toward the equivalent actor.

▪ Need for system level arbitration in the optimisation of safety strategies

▪ Need for simplification[1]

1 *Medicines, Management and Modernisation; a huge macabre Degeling et al.* 2003 in BMJ 326

2 Amalberti, in Press

Leadership

A great deal has been written about the role of leadership and its fundamental importance to achieving a successful change. Effective leadership can ensure that an organisation is effective, efficient and enabling. This is not a 'Taylorist' view of leadership with one leader and everyone else who simply follows. Such 'leaders' have the delusion of control but control very little. Ralph Stacey[1] says that organisations organise themselves. The key management ability is to participate in that process and to bring meaning and to champion quality. Unfortunately, when leaders lack the ability to give meaning or they experience difficulty, they often revert to micromanagement where process substitutes for vision.

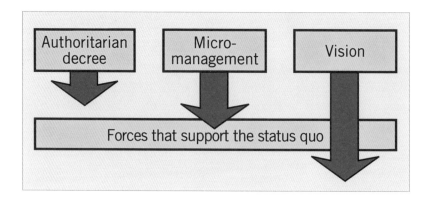

FIGURE 98
Breaking through
resistance to change

Kotter believes that issuing decrees and indulging in micromanagement are not effective and may even strengthen status quo. (Figure 98). Vision needs to be simply and constantly communicated and reinforced. The functions of leadership are contrasted with management as shown in figure 99. The message is that both leadership and management are necessary. One does not substitute for the other.

FIGURE 99
Leadership vs
Management functions

	Leadership Functions	Management Functions
Creating an agenda	*Establishes Direction: vision of the future, develops strategies for change to achieve goals.*	*Plans and Budgets: decides actions and timetables, allocates resources.*
Developing people	*Aligning People: communicates vision and strategy, influences creation of teams which accept the validity of the goals.*	*Organinsing and Staffing decides structure and allocates staff, develops policies, procedures and monitoring*
Execution	*Motivating and Inspiring: energises people to overcome obstacles, satisfies human needs*	*Controlling, Problem Solving: monitors results against plan and takes corrective action*
Outcome	*Produces positive and sometimes dramatic change*	*Produces order, consistancy and predictability*

1 *Strategic Management and Organisational Dynamics: the Challenge of complexity.* Stacey, 2003

Managers and Clinicians: A difficult relationship

Traditionally in the NHS, there is some division between the management of services and clinical aspects of care. Current knowledge suggests that this enables medical practitioners to focus on the patient, while managers deal with administration, providing an environment within which clinicians are able to work. Change projects can blur these boundaries, with management encroaching on clinical issues of priority.

Managing relationships with clinical staff is therefore a key element of any change programme. Conflict between the goals of an improvement project (improving services for all patients) and the goals of the clinician (doing the best for each patient as they present) can occur.

Alistair Mant in his book Intelligent Leadership[1], describes the relationship between managers and doctors as a clash between 'binary' and 'ternary' modes of thinking. In the binary mode of thought, someone always comes out on top. (Figure 100)

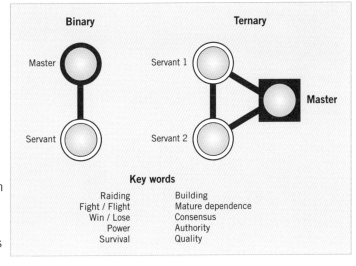

FIGURE 100
Binary and Ternary modes of behaviour (from Mant 1997, p6)[1]

This mode of behaviour is about winning, and both managers and doctors see the other as functioning in this way. However, each sees their own behaviour as operating in a ternary mode, where they are basing their decisions on some more worthy external reference point. Typically for doctors, the external higher purpose relates to patient care and the Hippocratic oath. For managers, the higher purpose relates to financial accountability and the 'greatest good for the greatest number'. Mant argues that as long as each see themselves as operating in a ternary fashion while seeing the other as operating in a binary fashion, no true dialogue can take place.

For improvement projects, a true partnership is necessary and what is needed is a way to break through this impasse. Mant suggests that the first step is to see the other party as operating in a ternary fashion, and then to identify the external reference point that they are using. While essentially administrative rather than patient care focussed, projects such the introduction of patient focussed booking challenge the right of medical staff to practice in the way they have in the past. They are seen by doctors as management intruding into areas of patient care, and will be resisted by medical staff unless the goal of the project can be related to their external reference point.

It is beholden on the manager wanting to make this sort of change to forge a partnership with clinicians. The first step is to always treat the medical staff as operating in a ternary fashion — never resorting to the 'difficult doctor' defence. The second is to do everything possible to ensure that the medical staff can perceive the ternary nature of your relationship with the problem.

1 *Intelligent Leadership.* Mant, 1997

FIGURE 101
The Doctor/Manager
relationship (from Mant
1997, p8)

'Intelligent Leadership'

Mant suggests that this can be done through the development of 'intelligent leadership'. Essentially, Mant's premise is that leadership by managers will only be successful if it is based on authority granted by the clinician to the manager. Authority will only be granted if it is based on a shared acceptance of common purpose (a shared ternary purpose) but especially if the clinician sees the manager as having a distinct contribution to the change process.

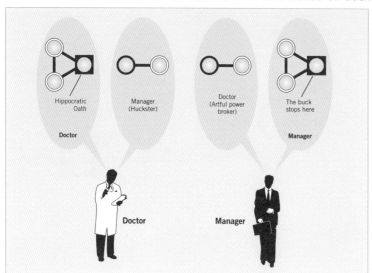

This often relates to skills held by the manager that the clinician does not have, but does value. In the context of Mant's approach, the challenge is to identify the 'intelligence' that can be brought to the relationship. Within the NHS, one key to this 'intelligence' can be the gathering and interpretation of data.

Leadership Styles

Mant (1997) also describes the 'optimum tripod of work' (figure 102) relating the feelings of those working in a system to the work environment or failure of managers. In the ideal state the manager tasks the subordinate clearly, stating not what needs to be done but rather what outputs are expected. The manager then trusts the subordinate to do the task, but maintains a minimally watchful position (tending), which Mant describes as 'appear(ing) at your shoulder just at the moment that you wish he or she would'. Mant suggests that this balance creates a learning environment which will develop staff potential, and increase the overall level of intelligence in the organisation.

He contrasts this optimal situation with the two 'out of balance' approaches. In the first of these, the rigid tripod (figure 103), managers do not trust staff, so the environment becomes one of policing rather than tasking.
The atmosphere will rapidly turn to one of paralysis and alienation, with staff showing little initiative because the environment does not allow for mistakes to be made.

In the second case, (figure 104) the environment is one of neglect. Mant sees this environment as a consequence of uninformed devolvement where there is unsupported (untended) handing over of accountability to staff unwilling or unable to cope with the additional responsibility. This lack of tending leads to ignorance and guesswork on the part of subordinates, and a climate of anomie.

Summary

- Change programmes can fail when there is insufficient planning. There are both process and people issues to consider.

- The prevailing organisational culture is fundamental to achieving successful and sustainable change where quality improvement becomes routine rather than project based.

- Myriad cultural reasons will resist change and seek to preserve the status quo. These can be personal, organisational, managerial or professional.

- Leadership which conveys vision and which enables people is the most effective way of developing a high service quality culture. It is far more effective than traditional models of control and micromanagement.

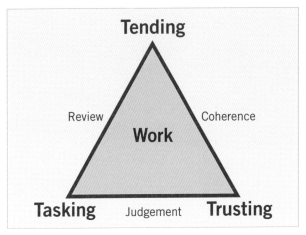

FIGURE 102
The optimum tripod of work

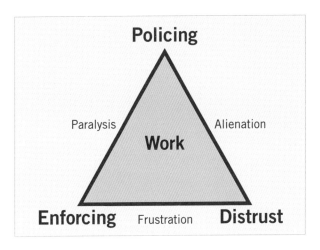

FIGURE 103
The rigid tripod of work

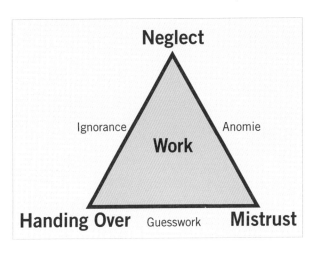

FIGURE 104
The diffuse tripod of work

9.2 Leadership and Culture   197

The human dimensions of change

No change can be achieved without the support of all those involved. There are a number of approaches to managing the human dimensions of change, and this is a brief introduction of some of the approaches to involving staff in the change process.

Most people do not like change, particularly when it is not their idea. Implementing change successfully inevitably means working with people who would prefer things to continue as they are. How is it possible to get people to not only cooperate with the change process, but to be enthusiastic about it?

Top down versus bottom up
Change can be imposed by management, or it can develop organically from below.

Top down change will usually have a clear plan, will have support and leadership, and will have clear objectives. On the other hand, staff will see the change process as imposition from above and they are less likely to feel part of the process.

Bottom up change will be more inclusive of staff, because this is change from 'within the ranks'. It is likely to be a continuous, rather than an episodic, process. There is often no plan or clear objective to the change. Outcomes may not be supported by senior management, as they may not fit with organisational objectives. There is less likely to be senior management acceptance of solutions.

The best option is a combination of the two approaches. Clear leadership and support for the process from management, with clear objectives. Staff should be using improvement tools in their daily work, and change should be a continuous process.

Change will be encouraged by 'intelligent leadership[1]'. Clinicians are more likely to become involved in change if they are confident that managers understand the problems faced by the service, and are competent in the analysis and understanding of data.

The four essential factors
Before staff will encompass change there are four factors that must be present.

Dissatisfaction
Staff must be unhappy with the process as it currently is. No one will want to change something that they think is working well.

1 *Intelligent Leadership.* Mant, 1997

Vision

There must be a view that things can be better, and an agreed vision of how things could be. We do not give up what we have without a clear idea of what we will put in its place.

Capacity

There must be capacity to change. There must be a commitment from management to the change process and to providing the resources that will be necessary to implement the change.

First steps

There must be a clear understanding by all of what will happen first. Overcoming inertia is easier if there is a clear plan, with manageable first steps.

FIGURE 105
Moving the zones

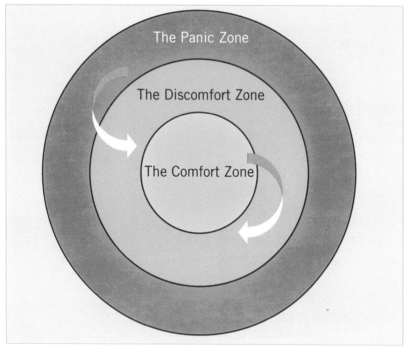

The Comfort Zone

Part of involving people is getting them out of that comfort zone where they feel that the status quo is OK. (Figure 105). But it must be done in such a way that staff do not panic. In any group there will be those in the comfort zone (I don't want to change), and those in the panic zone (I can't change). The art is in moving both into the discomfort zone (I can change).

What is in it for me?

The best way to move people is to identify what is in the change process for them. Everyone will have some motivation for either adopting or resisting change. Everyone will have something about the current process that they do not like. The key of good change management is to identify and use these drivers. Ensure that solutions to problems meet the needs of the staff, and they will be much easier to implement.

Transitions

'Every beginning ends something' — Paul Valery, French poet

Every change destroys something that has gone before, and some people will regret that loss even if they are happy with the new process.

William Bridges[1] calls the process that people go through as they face change 'transition'. Transitions start with an ending, go through a period of uncertainty, and end with a new beginning.

1 *Managing Transitions: Making the most of change.* Bridges, 1981

1. Managing the ending

Before you can start something new, you must end what used to be. To do this effectively you must understand who is losing what? What is over? You must positively acknowledge the losses and be clear what is over and what isn't.

It is often useful to ritually mark endings. In some cases, you can let people take a bit of the past with them — their door sign, their desk, a plant or poster.

2. Managing the neutral zone

Neither the old ways nor the new ways seem to be working. This is the dangerous time, where anxiety rises and motivation falls. There will be more illness, but it is also a more creative time — redefine it and use it constructively. Create temporary systems to manage through this stage.

3. A new beginning

This is the easy part, especially if the endings have been managed. You must clarify and communicate the purpose, painting a picture of how it will be. Create a plan, and show everyone their part in the future.

PDSA cycles: a model for improvement

After analysis, after identifying the problems, comes the moment of truth. What can be done to improve the service? How can changes be introduced in a clinical environment so that staff feel comfortable and patient care is improved not disrupted? Traditionally, the NHS approach to change has been through project management. Project plans are produced, Gantt charts prepared, programmes of meetings arranged. Change is introduced, but meets opposition and does not always succeed.

The NLIAH recommends an alternative approach to introducing change. A process of continuous improvement through incremental change, the use of PDSA cycles provides a model of improvement that enables an ongoing change programme to exist in a clinical environment.

What is the PDSA model?
The model for improvement has two parts: it starts with three questions, followed by a series of improvement cycles.

1. What are we trying to accomplish?
The start of the improvement process should be statement of the aims of the project. It is impossible to reach a goal without knowing what it is. The goal statement should be clear, specific, aspirational and measurable.

2. How will know that a change is an improvement?
The key to an effective improvement process is measurement. Without effective measures there is no way to know whether any change is improving the process. Selection of a range of measures for improvement should be central to any improvement process.

3. What changes can we make that will result in improvement?
PDSA cycles are a way of testing suggested improvements in a controlled environment. The changes that are developed in response to question 3 are the changes that the cycles will test. Changes can come from staff suggestion, from other sites who have looked at the same problems, or from the literature. The NLIAH has developed a database of good practice which can also be used as a source of ideas[1].

1 www.nliah.wales.nhs.uk

FIGURE 106
The PDSA cycle

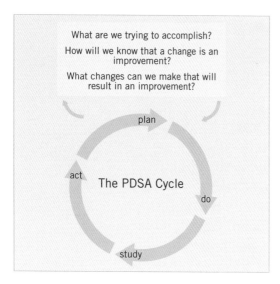

The PDSA Cycle
The PDSA cycle is a repeated cycle of four stages.
(Figure 106).

Plan
Define the question that you want answered in this cycle, including what you would expect the outcome to be expected. Design an experiment to test the question, covering the 'who, what, when and how' of the cycle, and the measures that will be used to determine success.

Do
Do the experiment, ensuring the data have been collected. Record what went wrong, and what went well. Were there any unexpected outcomes?

FIGURE 107
Improvement: A series of cycles

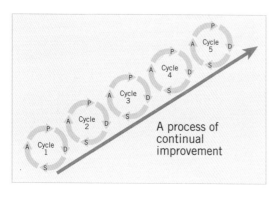

Study
Get everyone together to look at the data. What has been learned? Do the outcomes agree with the predictions? Are there circumstances where the outcome might be different?

Act
Decide what to do in the next cycle. Should the change be implemented more widely? Can it be extended to more patients, or is something else necessary? What will be the objective of the next cycle? If the change was unsuccessful, it should be abandoned and something different tried for the next cycle — there should not be pressure to adopt every change.

FIGURE 108
A recording form

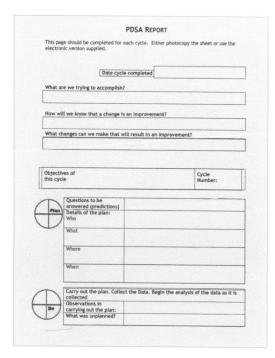

A series of cycles
Improvement is the result of a continual series of cycles building on previous results. Each PDSA cycle is short, making small improvements to the status quo. The result is a steady improvement in process over time. One 'ramp' of cycles relating to one process may be undertaken in parallel with another series dealing with a different problem, but the key is to have a series of changes, made in a systematic fashion, with evidence of the results from each cycle, over a period of time.

Advantages of PDSA
The PDSA model is ideally suited to introducing change in a complex clinical environment, where there is a high element of risk. Small changes are more acceptable to staff and patients, and there is far less disruption than the more traditional 'major redesign programme'. The process also promotes the philosophy that change is a normal continuous process that the staff are involved in, rather than a major event that 'happens' to people.

GP feedback systems

When talking to consultants and GPs about direct access to outpatient appointments, two things become clear. Consultants are concerned about the number of referrals wrongly directed, with inadequate information, uncompleted tests, or wrongly prioritised. GPs are concerned about receiving feedback on the quality of, or problems with, referrals. There should be a process to address these concerns. The NLIAH recommends the following approach.

The best way to monitor and regulate any process is through the provision of good information, and in particular, the presence of formal feedback loops. Despite this, there is still a lack of meaningful feedback between secondary care and primary care about the process of referral (as opposed to the outcome of the referral). Instead, there is a tendency for secondary care to attempt to 'control' the referral process by imposing referral guidelines, a process that has been tried for years with a singular lack of success.

There is a place for referral guidance from secondary care – the 'Medic to Medic©' approach adopted by Conwy and Denbighshire NHS Trust is one such system. Yet guidelines alone will not change behaviour. The NLIAH suggests the following process.

Step 1

Guidelines are either developed by a working party of GPs and consultants, or adapted from another source. While it is unlikely that every GP and consultant will be involved in writing the guidelines, it is important to get as many involved as possible if the guidelines are going to be accepted by the primary care community.

Step 2

Using clinical guidelines, the GP determines if the patient requires a referral to secondary care. The guidelines should be simply that – guidelines. They should not be prescriptive, and should not prevent the GP from referring a patient about whose care they are concerned, even if that patient falls outside the guidelines. This is particularly important if the guidelines are computerised, as some computer based systems will not allow a referral outside the guidelines to be made. Guidelines are never a substitute for clinical judgement.

FIGURE 109
Flowchart of the GP
feedback system

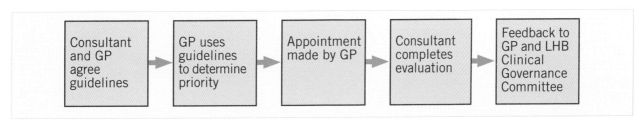

The GP will also make an assessment of the urgency attached to the referral, and the appropriate destination of the referral (generic referral, or to a specific consultant, or is this patient best seen by another member of the clinical team?)

An appointment is made as a result of the referral process, and the patient attends the appointment. As this is the first time that the Consultant has had a chance to evaluate the 'appropriateness' of the referral, urgency and destination of the referral, this is the point at which an evaluation should be completed (not, as is often the case, when the referral letter is seen by the consultant.)

As part of the outpatient appointment, therefore, an evaluation form should be completed. This form (a sample can be seen in figure 110) should be computer-generated from the PAS, and should be as administratively simple to complete as possible. The aim of the form should be to provide good feedback to the GP, while not taking additional time in the clinic to complete. The default condition, requiring no more than a tick or signature, should be that all was well with the referral.

The evaluation form is returned to the GP, either directly from the clinic, or with the patient letter generated at the outpatient appointment. This will provide the GP with specific feedback about the referral, and will inform their behaviour on future occasions.

What happens if there are specific 'problems' with referrals?

This process provides feedback to the GP about the process of their referral. Because each event is treated as 'one-off' this process alone will not identify specific referral problems across a population of GPs. To achieve this, an additional process is required. In some form, data should be collected from the evaluation forms and stored to identify educational requirements. To reduce the administrative load that this process could create, machine-readable forms could be used.

There are two ways in which this aggregated data may be useful.

1 Identifying education needs of the GP community

There may be specific conditions that generate poor referrals across many GPs. This could be caused by a misconception within the wider GP community of the appropriate urgency of a certain condition; by a change in practice such that certain conditions could be managed in primary care yet GPs are not yet aware of the change; or changes in the Trust that means that certain categories of referrals are now more appropriately sent to other clinicians. If some basic data from the evaluation forms is entered into database, problem referrals for specific conditions could indicate a specific education need which can then be addressed by the Trust, improving the referral process for the GP, the Trust and the patient.

FIGURE 110
Feedback form

2 Issues with specific GPs

There may also be cases where aggregated data identify issues with specific GPs. With the agreement of the GP and Local Health Board, summary information could be sent to the LHB clinical governance committee. This committee should have the responsibility of addressing issues of poor referral behaviour by specific GPs or practices. This is not an issue that the Trust should deal with themselves. There may however be an education role for the Trust at the LHB's request.

The intention of a feedback process is to improve the referral process both for the GP and the patient, and to reduce the unnecessary work within the Trust redirecting appointments, or seeing patients best treated in some other way. For this reason, the benefits of the process must outweigh the administrative costs associated with it. It is vital that in generating the forms in clinic and in entering the data into a database, the system be as simple as possible, with the bulk of forms needing no intervention. For this reason, there may be a tendency to only 'fill out the problems', and ignoring the bulk of 'good' referrals. There is a risk to this approach, as there is value in positive feedback, and a system that only generates feedback when there are problems will be less supported by primary care.

Secondary care often complains about referrals: trusts want 'demand management', GPs want speedy service. A process of effective and reasonable feedback, with links into the clinical governance and educational processes, will meet the needs of all parties in the process.

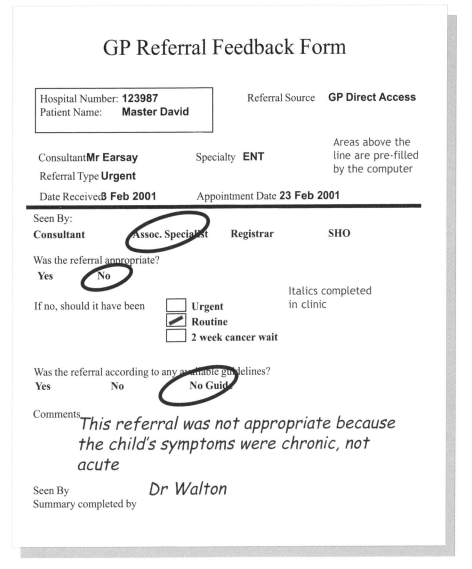

GP Referral Feedback Form

Hospital Number: **123987**
Patient Name: **Master David**

Referral Source **GP Direct Access**

Consultant **Mr Earsay**   Specialty **ENT**

Referral Type **Urgent**

Areas above the line are pre-filled by the computer

Date Received **8 Feb 2001**   Appointment Date **23 Feb 2001**

Seen By:

Consultant   Assoc. Specialist   Registrar   SHO

Was the referral appropriate?

Yes   No

If no, should it have been

☐ **Urgent**
☑ **Routine**
☐ **2 week cancer wait**

Italics completed in clinic

Was the referral according to any available guidelines?
Yes   No   No Guide

Comments *This referral was not appropriate because the child's symptoms were chronic, not acute*

Seen By   *Dr Walton*
Summary completed by

Useful resources

This document provides a very brief introduction to a number of different tools and techniques. It is hoped that the following resources will allow you to delve deeper into some of the tools and learning resources.

A good starting place for more information is the National Leadership and Innovation Agency for Healthcare website: www.nliah.wales.nhs.uk

Government Publications

Designed for Life: Creating world class Health and Social Care for Wales in the 21st Century
Welsh Assembly Government, 2005.

Improving the Health in Wales: A Guide for the NHS with its Partners
Welsh Assembly Government, 2001.

The Review of Health and Social Care in Wales
Report of the Project Team advised by Derek Wanless.
Welsh Assembly Government, 2003.

Waiting List Accuracy: Assessing the Accuracy of Waiting List Information in NHS Hospitals in England and Wales
The Audit Commission, 2003.

Audit Commission Acute Hospital Portfolio Report on Operating Theatres
The Audit Commission, 2003.

NHS Waiting Times in Wales
Report by the National Audit Office Wales on behalf of the Auditor General for Wales, 2005. ISBN 1-90-421925-X

Copying Letters to Patients: Summaries of 12 Pilot Project Sites
Health Organisations Research Centre, Manchester School of Management, 2003.

A Guide to Good Practice: Day Surgery in Wales
Innovations in Care, Welsh Assembly Government, 2004. ISBN 0750435151

A Guide to Good Practice: Integrated Care Pathways
National Leadership & Innovation Agency for Healthcare, 2005.
ISBN 1-905456-01-8

Healthcare Improvement

To Err is Human: Building a safer health system
Institute of Medicine Report, 2000. ISBN 0309068371

Crossing the Quality Chasm
Institute of Medicine Report, 2001. ISBN 0309072808

Curing Healthcare. New Strategies for Quality Improvement
Donald M Berwick, A Blanton Godfrey, Jane Roessner, 1990.
ISBN 0787964522

Escape Fire. Designs for the Future of Health Care
Donald M Berwick, 2004. ISBN 0787972177

Modernisation Agency Publications
A complete list of Modernisation Agency Publications can be obtained from
their website: www.content.modern.nhs.uk

Modernisation Agency: Improvement Leaders Guide Updated Boxed Set
12 separate guides available as boxed set. Modernisation Agency, 2005

10 High Impact Changes for Service Improvement and Delivery
Modernisation Agency, 2004.

Quality Improvement
The Improvement Guide: A Practical Approach to Enhancing Organisational
Performance
Langley, Nolan, Nolan, Norman & Provost, 1997. ISBN 0787902578

Quality Improvement Through Planned Experimentation
Moen, Nolan, & Provost, 1999. ISBN 0-07-913781-4

The Fifth Discipline: The Art and Practice of the Learning Organisation
Peter Senge, 1993. ISBN 0712656871

The Fifth Discipline Fieldbook
Peter Senge, 1994. ISBN 1857880609

The Dance of Change: The Challenges of Sustaining Momentum in a
Learning Organisation (a Fifth Discipline Resource)
Peter Senge, 1999. ISBN 1857882431

Understanding Variation: The Key to Managing Chaos (2nd Edition)
Donald J Wheeler, 2000. ISBN 0945320531

The Memory Jogger Plus+ and Featuring the Seven Management and
Planning Tools
Michael Brassard, 1989. ISBN 1879364417.

Promoting Advanced Access in Primary Care: A handbook
Thomas S Warrender, 2002. ISBN 1902115252.

Lean Thinking: Banish Waste and Create Wealth in Your Corporation (revised)
James P Womack and Daniel T Jones, 2003. ISBN 0743249275

The Lean Toolbox.
John Bicheno, 2000. ISBN 0951382993

Presenting Information
Visual Explanations: Images and Quantities, Evidence and Narrative
Edward R Tufte, 1997. ISBN 0961392126

The Visual Display of Quantitative Information
Edward R Tufte, 2002. ISBN 0961392142

Envisioning Information
Edward R Tufte, 1990. ISBN 0961392118

Leadership Skills

Intelligent Leadership
Alistair Mant, 1999. ISBN 1865080527

Leading Change
John P Kotter, 1996. ISBN 0875847471

Managing Transitions: Making Sense of Life's Changes
William Bridges, 1981. ISBN 0201000822

Improvement, Trust and Healthcare Workforce.
*Donald Berwick, 2003, Quality and Safety in Healthcare v12
supplement1 pp2-6.*

The leader's digest: timeless principles for team and organisation success.
J Clemmer, 2003. ISBN 0968467512

Medicines, management and modernisation, a huge macabre?
P Degeling, S Maxwell, J Kennedy, B Coyle, 2003, BMJ 326: 649-652

Influencing sceptical staff to become supporters of service improvement:
a qualitative study of doctors' and managers' views.
*Gollop R, Whitby E, Buchanan D, Ketley D, 2004,
Quality and Safety in Healthcare v13 no2 p108-114.*

Diffusion of innovations in service organizations: systematic review and
recommendations
*Greenhalgh T and MacFarlane F., 2004 in Health Management:
The Journal for Health Management in the NHS and the Independent Sector*

Great Boss, Dead Boss
Ray Immelmon, 2003. ISBN 0974036919

Strategic Management and organisational dynamics:
the challenge of complexity
R D Stacey, 2003, 4th edition. ISBN 027364212X

Theatre specific information

National Good Practice Guidance on Pre-operative Assessment for Day Surgery
Modernisation Agency, 2002.

National Good Practice Guidance on Pre-operative Assessment for inpatients
Modernisation Agency, 2003.

Pre-operative Assessment: The Role of the Anaesthetist
The Association of Anaesthetists of Great Britain and Ireland, 2001.

Good Practice in Consent Implementation Guide: Consent to examination
or treatment
Welsh Assembly Government, 2002.

The Perioperative System: A New Approach to Managing Elective Surgery
R Kerridge, A Lee, E Latchford, S J Beehan, K M Hillman, 1995.
Anaesthesia and Intensive Care, Vol.23, No. 5

Development and Effectiveness of an Anaesthesia Preoperative Evaluation
Clinic in a Teaching Hospital
S Fischer, 1996. Anesthesiology, Vol. 85, No.1

The Theory of Constraints, and Critical Chain Project Management

The Goal
Eliyahu M Goldratt, Jeff Cox, 1989. ISBN 0884270610

It's Not Luck
Eliyahu M Goldratt, 2002. ISBN 0566076276

Critical Chain
Eliyahu M Goldratt, 1997. ISBN 0884271536

Necessary but Not Sufficient: A Theory of Constraints Business Novel
Eliyahu M Goldratt, Eli Schragenheim, Carol A Ptak,2000 . ISBN 0884271706

Project Management in the Fast Lane: Applying the Theory of Constraints
Robert C Newbold, 1998. ISBN 1574441957

Goldratt's Theory of Constraints: A Systems Approach to
Continuous Improvement
H William Dettmer, 1998. ISBN 0873893700

What is this Thing Called the Theory of Constraints and
How Should it be Implemented
Eliyahu M Goldratt, 1994. ISBN 0884270858

The Haystack Syndrome: Sifting Information out of the Data Ocean
Eliyahu M Goldratt, 1991 . ISBN 0884270890

Deming and Goldratt: The Theory of Constraints and the System of
Profound Knowledge
D. Lepore and O Cohen, 1999. ISBN 0884271633

Management Dilemmas: The Theory of the Constraint Approach to
Problem Identification and Solutions
Eli Schragenheim, 1998. ISBN 1574442228

The Measurement Nightmare: How the theory of Constraints can
Resolve Conflicting Strategies, Policies, and Measures
Debra Smith, 1999. ISBN 1574442465

Critical Chain Project Management
Lawrence P Leach, 2000. ISBN 1580530745.

The definitive guide to project management: the fast-track to getting the job
done on time and on budget
*Sebastian Nokes, Ian Major, Alan Greenwood, Dominic Allen and
Mark Goodman, 2003. ISBN 0273663976*

Websites

www.nliah.wales.nhs.uk
The website of the National Leadership and Innovation Agency for Healthcare.

www.content.modern.nhs.uk
This is the website of the English NHS Modernisation Agency, and provides a gateway to all their other sites and documents.

www.ihi.org
The Institute of Healthcare Improvement website.

www.dh.gov.uk
The Department Health in England Website, giving access to good practice guidelines for "copying letters to patients" in England, and the Waiting, Booking and Choice programme website.

www.audit-commission.gov.uk
The Audit Commission website.

www.nice.org.uk
The National Institute for Clinical Excellence website.

www.his.org.uk
The Hospital Infection Society website

www.afpp.org.uk
the Association for Perioperative Practice (AfPP) incorporating NATN (The National Association of Theatre Nurses)

www.aodp.org
The Association of Operating Department Practitioners.

www.cf.ac.uk/carbs/lerc
The Lean Enterprise Resource Centre at Cardiff University.

www.bmj.bmjjournals.com
Access to the British Medical Journal.

www.qhc.bmjjournals.com
Access to the journal Quality and Safety in Healthcare.

www.lean.org
The official website of the Lean Enterprise Institute.

www.goldratt.co.uk
The official Goldratt UK website.

www.jeantodd.co.uk.
The Jean Todd Partnership (Appointment Centre training).

www.juran.com
The site of the Juran Institute, a Continuous Quality Improvement trainer and resources site

www.brecker.com/quality.htm
Another Continuous Quality Improvement movement site, using the work of Deming and Juran.

www.galileoinitiative.com
A change management organisation

www.ihm.org.uk
The Institute of Healthcare Management website

www.qbq.com
The site of The Question Behind the Question, a quality improvement organisation